The Handbook of
Psychiatric Drugs

The Handbook of

Psychiatric Drugs

A CONSUMER'S GUIDE TO SAFE AND EFFECTIVE USE

Second Edition

Bernard Salzman, M.D., D.A.B.P.N.

An Owl Book

Henry Holt and Company   New York

Henry Holt and Company, Inc.
Publishers since 1866
115 West 18th Street
New York, New York 10011

Henry Holt® is a registered
trademark of Henry Holt and Company, Inc.

Published in Canada by Fitzhenry & Whiteside Ltd.,
195 Allstate Parkway, Markham, Ontario L3R 4T8.

Library of Congress Cataloging-in-Publication Data
Salzman, Bernard.
The handbook of psychiatric drugs: a consumer's guide to safe
and effective use / Bernard Salzman.—2nd ed.
p.   cm.
"An Owl book."
Includes index.
1. Psychotropic drugs—Handbooks, manuals, etc.
2. Consumer education.   I. Title.
RM315.S22   1996   96-5229
615'.78—dc20   CIP

ISBN 0-8050-4468-X

Henry Holt books are available for special promotions
and premiums. For details contact: Director, Special Markets.

First Edition—1991
Second Edition—1996

Printed in the United States of America
All first editions are printed on acid-free paper. ∞

1   3   5   7   9   10   8   6   4   2

The information in this book was designed to educate individuals on some of the effects and uses of psychiatric medication. It is in no way meant as a substitute for regular medical and/or psychiatric care. The author strongly recommends that the drugs profiled herein be used only under the supervision of a psychiatrist or other medical doctor.

To my wife—the secret courier—who suffered and prompted this author throughout the entire process. And to my three children, to whom I owe far more than has been written or spoken.

Acknowledgments

I would like to express my appreciation to John Gallagher, without whom this book would not have been possible; his considerable writing skills made it a reality. I would also like to thank my editor at Henry Holt, Theresa Burns, who originally proposed the idea for this book and whose patience and editorial skills were sorely needed at times.

I would also like to acknowledge my patients, past and present. In many respects, they were and are my true teachers. These good people taught me patience, empathy, and most of all, the need and ability to listen.

Contents

Contents

Introduction

This is a handbook for people who take psychiatric drugs—also known as *designer* drugs or *mood* drugs. Although some of these labels imply something exotic, or even enjoyable, the function of these drugs is really quite soberingly simple. Millions of us use them on a temporary basis to alleviate depression, combat anxiety, and help us sleep. For some, they can mean the difference between functioning normally on a daily basis or remaining incapacitated by a psychiatric disorder. Like all medications, they work only when used properly by people who understand their limitations as well as their potential. And so this book is also about the relationship between you and these drugs, how they can be used safely and with the most benefit to you.

Fifty years ago, we usually institutionalized people suffering from chronic manic-depression or psychotic episodes. The more agitated ones were heavily sedated, and often received the relatively new treatment of *electroconvulsive therapy* (ECT), otherwise known as shock therapy.

At that time, some of the other psychiatric treatments available and commonly used included *hydrotherapy*, in which the patient was immersed in hot baths and swaddled in towels; *insulin shock,* a process designed to make someone so hypoglycemic that seizures were induced; and *barbiturates*, the primary psychiatric drug of its day, used to sedate or, in effect, to incapacitate the agitated individual. Certainly we were in the early stages of our understanding of the brain and how it functions, especially with regard to psychological behaviors.

Since that time, most of the advances made in the treatment of psychiatric disorders involve new medications. As so often happens with scientific discoveries, the development of many of these new drugs was linked to chance discoveries. Perhaps the best example occurred about forty years ago when doctors noted that many of their patients with tuberculosis seemed unusually happy even though faced with what was then a universally grave, often fatal disease: consumption. What set these people apart from other patients was the fact that they were all being treated with a new antitubercular drug called iproniazid. The significance of this drug-related euphoria was not lost on the biochemists of the day. Research into the particular properties of iproniazid led to the eventual development of several related drugs that are now used for mood elevation. One of those drugs became the first of the tricyclic antidepressants, imipramine (see page 99).

Our progress in the treatment of psychiatric illnesses is also linked to our growing understanding of the brain itself. About twenty years ago we discovered the existence of specific receptor sites in the brain that are host to a number of brain chemicals called *neurotransmitters*. Once we began to understand, in part, the function of these chemical messengers, researchers were able to develop specific medications that either imitated their effects or altered their action.

Over the next five to ten years (in the 1990s), as we come to understand more about how the brain functions, we are sure to discover still newer drugs that will act more efficiently and with fewer side effects than those we currently use.

I entered into this story of behavior and treatment about twenty-five years ago when I began my medical training at Bellevue Hospital in New York City, an institution with a long historical relationship with the mentally ill. The mid-1960s was also a time in which the public attitude toward the *recreational* use of prescriptive and illicit mind-expanding drugs underwent a dramatic change. As a result, these drugs were widely used with absolutely disastrous results. In the emergency room at Bellevue, I saw hundreds of people admitted with a variety of psychiatric disorders, including acute drug reactions. Many were my own age and more than of few of them died. By the end of my residency, I had received a sobering education—and it was not the last one—in the human damage caused by drug abuse.

Following my residency, I served as the drug-abuse expert for the 13th Air Force as part of my tour of duty in Southeast Asia. As head of their mental-hygiene clinic, I treated scores of men, especially those returning from Vietnam, who had a variety of serious health-care problems, all directly or indirectly related to their abuse of drugs.

Serving in a war zone where there were few enforceable regulations concerning the use of drugs, I saw many young men develop drug habits, particularly for marijuana, amphetamines, heroin, and barbiturates. As the drug problem became more serious and widespread, I was asked to travel to different Air Force squadrons throughout the Philippines and talk to servicemen about the pitfalls of drug abuse.

When I returned to Bellevue Hospital, I founded a new drug treatment program, the first *dual diagnosis* program in the world: the psychiatric treatment of severely disturbed patients who were also heroin addicts.

In the early days of methadone treatment, people with severe psychiatric disorders were excluded from drug rehabilitation with methadone, since the hospital wanted to demonstrate the effectiveness of the drug on a more reliable patient. Heroin addicts with severe psychiatric disorders were thought to be less controllable, less predictable, less compliant. Conventional medical opinion at the time held that these people would only misuse conventional psychiatric drugs—just as they had misused other drugs.

The new program I was setting up departed from traditional

medical thinking since it intended to treat the addict's psychiatric disorder with psychiatric drugs, many of which were known to be potentially habit-forming.

Over time, the program permitted us to treat people in a way that recognized both their problems with drug dependence and also their need for conventional psychiatric medications. The success of psychiatric drugs such as THORAZINE helped many addicts not only control and manage their underlying psychiatric disorder, but also their dependence on heroin. We were thus able to make respectable the safe and effective use of conventional psychiatric drugs for drug-dependent individuals.

In 1979, I became a Senior Consultant to the Division of Drug Rehabilitation, as well as a Chief of Adult Inpatient Services at Bellevue, a more conventional medical service that treats patients with a variety of psychiatric illnesses. For the past twenty years, in my private practice I have also treated hundreds of individuals who suffered from both drug-misuse problems and conventional psychiatric illnesses, such as depression, anxiety, and psychosis.

In many ways my professional career has been devoted to educating the medical community not only on the treatability of individuals with drug abuse problems, but also on the psychology and philosophy of drug therapy. Both as a current faculty member of the New York University Medical School and as a lecturer at graduate schools both in the United States and Europe, I have found that the issues surrounding the use of drugs among people who abuse drugs and those who do not are remarkably similar. Both groups are often uninformed or sadly misinformed.

Admittedly, drug abuse is a psychologically, sociologically, and philosophically complicated problem. But if we want health-care professionals to develop humane and effective drug-treatment programs, as well as to empower individuals to use psychiatric drugs responsibly, education must continue to play a major role. Among the many matters I discuss with my patients before prescribing psychiatric drugs are: the importance of those situations in their lives that predictably lead to drug interactions, why a respect for latency and washout periods can reduce the possibility of drug misuse, and how strict adherence to agreed-upon drug schedules and proper termination procedures are central to a successful outcome.

That is why, in this handbook, I have presented information on these issues *before* profiling the drugs themselves in Chapter 6. Although I am aware that most individuals do not read reference books like novels—that is, from beginning to end—my hope is that you will read this book as it has been organized here. If you were my patient and I were treating you personally, I would want you to be aware of all the considerations involved in the use of these drugs *before* I prescribed a single pill. This may mean some repetition from chapter to chapter, but the business of taking psychiatric drugs is a serious one, and anything that so directly affects our minds and our bodies is surely worth hearing more than once.

And so, in a spirit of respect for both the strengths and limitations of psychiatric medications, as well as the value of your own personal health, I hope you will read and take to heart the information found in this book.

BERNARD SALZMAN, M.D., D.A.B.P.N.

List of Psychiatric Drugs

FIRST-GENERATION TRICYCLICS

Brand Name	*Generic Name*
ELAVIL, ENDEP, EMITRIP, AMITRIL	amitriptyline (a-mee-TRIP-ti-leen)
TOFRANIL, TOFRANIL-PM, JANIMINE, TIPRAMINE	imipramine (im-IP-ra-meen)

SECOND-GENERATION TRICYCLICS

Brand Name	*Generic Name*
NORPRAMIN, PERTOFRANE	desipramine (dess-IP-ra-meen)
PAMELOR, AVENTYL	nortriptyline (nor-TRIP-ti-leen)
VIVACTIL, NEOACTIL	protriptyline (pro-TRIP-ti-leen)
SURMONTIL	trimipramine (trye-MIP-ra-meen)
ASENDIN	amoxapine (a-MOX-a-peen)
SINEQUAN, ADAPIN	doxepin (DOX-e-pin)
WELLBUTRIN	bupropion HCI (boo-PRO-pi-un)

SEROTONIN REUPTAKE BLOCKERS

Brand Name	*Generic Name*
DESYREL	trazodone (TRAZ-o-done)
PROZAC	fluoxetine (floo-OX-i-teen)
ANAFRANIL	clomipramine (klo-MIP-ra-meen)
LUVOX	fluvoxamine (floo-VOX-a-meen)
LUDIOMIL	maprotiline (ma-PRO-ti-leen)
EFFEXOR	venlafaxine (ven-la-FAX-een)
ZOLOFT	sertraline (SER-tra-leen)
PAXIL	paroxetine (pair-o-SET-een)
SERZONE	nefazadone (ne-FAZ-a-doan)

MONOAMINE-OXIDASE INHIBITORS

Brand Name	*Generic Name*
NARDIL	phenelzine (FEN-el-zeen)
MARPLAN	isocarboxazid (eye-so-kar-BOX-a-zid)
PARNATE	tranylcypromine (tran-ill-SIP-ro-meen)
EUTONYL	pargyline (PAR-gi-leen)
ELDEPRYL	selegiline (sell-e-GILL-een)

AUGMENTATION

Brand Name	*Generic Name*
LIMBITROL, LIMBITROL-DS	chlordiazepoxide (klor-dye-az-e-POX-ide) and amitriptyline (a-mee-TRIP-ti-leen)

THYROID HORMONE
LITHIUM
PSYCHOSTIMULANTS

ANTIPSYCHOTICS

LOW-POTENCY

Brand Name	*Generic Name*
THORAZINE	chlorpromazine (klor-PRO-ma-zeen)

Brand Name	Generic Name
MELLARIL, MILLAZINE	thioridazine (thye-oh-RID-a-zeen)
SERENTIL	mesoridazine (mez-o-RID-a-zeen)

HIGH-POTENCY

Brand Name	Generic Name
HALDOL	haloperidol (hey-lo-PAIR-ee-doll)
TRILAFON	perphenazine (per-FEN-a-zeen)
STELAZINE, SUPRAZINE	trifluoperazine (tri-FLOO-oh-pair-a-zeen)
NAVANE	thiothixene (thye-oh-THIX-een)
PROLIXIN, PERMITIL	fluphenazine (floo-FEN-a-zeen)
MOBAN	molindone (MO-lin-down)
LOXITANE	loxapine (LOX-a-peen)
COMPAZINE	prochlorperazine (pro-klor-PAIR-a-zeen)
ORAP	pimozide (PIM-oh-zide)
CLOZARIL	clozapine (KLAS-a-peen)

DEPOT

Brand Name	Generic Name
PROLIXIN	fluphenazine (floo-FEN-a-zeen) decanoate and fluphenazine enanthate
HALDOL	haloperidol (hey-lo-PAIR-ee-doll) decanoate
RISPERIDOL	risperidone (ris-PAIR-e-doan)

GATEWAY DRUGS

ANTI-CRAVING AGENT

Brand Name	Generic Name
REVIA	naltrexone (nal-TRECKS-zone)

COGNITIVE ENHANCEMENT AGENT

Brand Name	Generic Name
COGNEX	tacrine (TA-kreen)

HYPNOTIC SEDATIVES

BARBITURATES

Brand Name	Generic Name
AMYTAL	amobarbital (am-o-BAR-bi-tal)
SECONAL	secobarbital (see-ko-BAR-bi-tal)
NEMBUTAL	pentobarbital (pen-toe-BAR-bi-tal)
AMBIEN	zolpidem (zol-PEE-dem)

NONBARBITURATES

Brand Name	Generic Name
NOCTEC	chloral hydrate (klor-al HY-drate)
NOLUDAR, AQUACHLORAL SUPPRETTES	methyprylon (meth-i-PRYE-lon)
PLACIDYL	ethchlorvynol (eth-klor-VI-nole)
DORIDEN	glutethimide (gloo-TETH-i-mide)
VALMID	ethinamate (e-THIN-a-mate)
PARAL	paraldehyde (par-AL-de-hide)

BENZODIAZEPINES

Brand Name	Generic Name
DALMANE	flurazepam (flure-AZ-e-pam)
RESTORIL, RAZEPAM	temazepam (tem-AZ-e-pam)
HALCION	triazolam (trye-AY-zoe-lam)
DORAL	quazepam (GWA-zee-pam)

ANTIHISTAMINES

Brand Name	Generic Name
BENADRYL	diphenhydramine (dee-fen-HYE-dra-meen)
PHENERGAN	promethazine (pro-METH-a-zeen)
ATARAX, ANXAMIL, ATOZINE, DURRAX, E-VISTA, HYDROXACEN, HYZINE, QUIESS, VISTACON, VISTAJET, VISTAQUEL, VISTARIL, VISTAZINE	hydroxyzine (hy-DROX-i-zeen)

ANTIDYSKINETICS

Brand Name	Generic Name
ARTANE, TRIHEXANE, TRIHEXY	trihexyphenidyl (try-hex-e-FEN-i-dill)
SYMMETREL	amantadine (a-MAN-ta-deen)
COGENTIN	benztropine (BENZ-tro-peen)

PSYCHOSTIMULANTS

Brand Name	Generic Name
DEXEDRINE	dextroamphetamine (dex-tro-am-FET-a-meen)
RITALIN	methylphenidate (meth-ill-FEN-i-date)
CYLERT	pemoline (PEM-o-lin)
PONDIMIN	fenfluramine (fen-FLURE-a-meen)

ANTIANXIETY AGENTS

LONG-ACTING BENZODIAZEPINES

Brand Name	Generic Name
VALIUM	diazepam (dye-AZ-e-pam)
LIBRIUM	chlordiazepoxide (klor-dye-az-e-POX-ide)

PRO DRUGS

Brand Name	Generic Name
TRANXENE	chlorazepate (klor-AZ-e-pate) dipotassium
CENTRAX	prazepam (PRAZ-e-pam)
PAXIPAM	halazepam (hal-AZ-e-pam)

SHORT-ACTING BENZODIAZEPINES

Brand Name	Generic Name
XANAX	alprazolam (al-PRAZ-oh-lam)
ATIVAN, LORAZ, ALZAPEM	lorazepam (lor-AZ-e-pam)
SERAX	oxazepam (ox-AZ-e-pam)

SHORT-ACTING NONSPECIFIC

Brand Name	Generic Name
INDERAL	propranolol (pro-PRAN-oh-lol)
CATAPRES	clonidine (KLOE-ni-deen)
BUSPAR	buspirone (BOOS-peer-rown)

OBSOLETE DRUGS

Brand Name	Generic Name
EQUANIL, MILTOWN, MEPROSPAN, NEURAMATE, SEDABAMATE, TRANMEP	meprobamate (me-pro-BA-mate)

MOOD STABILIZERS

Brand Name	Generic Name
LITHIUM CARBONATE	lithium (LITH-e-oom)

LITHIUM SUBSTITUTES

Brand Name	Generic Name
TEGRETOL	carbamazepine (kar-ba-MAZ-e-peen)
DEPAKENE	valproic (val-PRO-ic) acid
KLONOPIN	clonazepam (clo-NAZ-e-pam)

ONE

What You Need to Know Before Taking Psychiatric Medications

The reasons people come to a psychiatrist range from the trivial to the life-threatening. With the help of various therapies and the judicious use of medicines, psychiatric treatment is capable of helping more and more people. However, many people feel ambivalent about seeking this kind of health care. Just the sound of the term *mental illness* still carries with it a taboo.

Distrust of Psychiatrists

Most of us share a cultural reluctance about revealing what really troubles us, especially those inner secrets and weaknesses to someone who is little more than a stranger—even if that person may be a doctor. In effect, going to a psychiatrist makes public that which

Note: In this discussion, I primarily use the term *psychiatrist* rather than *psychologist,* or *psychotherapy,* because many of my patients have told me they usually associate the term *psychiatric treatment* with more serious behavioral problems or symptoms and, consequently, the use of psychiatric drugs. I suspect this bias also exists outside my patient population.

many of us would prefer to hide or deny. It is an admission that we cannot control our personal problems. A cruel and false implication many of us share is that these kinds of problems stem from an emotional weakness which a stronger (read *better*) person would have solved without outside help. People suffering from alcoholism are often, for instance, faulted as people of weak character rather than seen as people who are caught up in the throes of a complicated disease that has profound psychological roots.

Another problem is what people expect from a psychiatrist. Many people come to me with a single model of what treatment will involve, usually drawn from conventional medicine. They expect that a psychiatric diagnosis and treatment will be as systematic and precise as that of most physical diseases. For example, when I ask some of my patients what they expect the therapeutic process will be all about, they tell me that they anticipate a period of talking therapy, after which they hope to receive from me an insight or explanation for their symptoms or behavior. At this point, they expect their therapy will lead to an orderly, if not prompt, cure.

Unfortunately, the psychotherapeutic treatment model differs in many respects from this understanding.

A common misunderstanding about expectations occurs when a person comes in looking for a cure for his or her insomnia and anxiety. She or he has been troubled by these symptoms for at least a month and maybe as long as six months or more. Early in our therapy, I may discover that these symptoms are related to a deeper underlying disorder, in this case possibly a depressive illness. As in conventional medicine, this person would be treated for both the symptoms and the underlying disease—the insomnia and anxiety *and* the depression.

For some people, however, an acknowledgment that depression may be the underlying problem causing their insomnia poses a more serious difficulty. They may be willing to accept simple help, especially in the form of a drug, to sleep well again; what they cannot accept is a deeper, perhaps darker, cause for their sleeplessness. Part of the problem is that unlike having an infection, which most people view as something that can come upon anyone, people with insomnia somehow feel responsible for *contracting* an underlying psychiatric illness, such as depression.

In addition to an unwillingness to expose what they would prefer to keep hidden, some people are afraid that I, or some other therapist, will be able to read their mind. They dread the idea that they would be unable to conceal or protect the source of their greatest shame(s), even though disclosure is what can lead to successful treatment. First I try to reassure them—by telling them that I *cannot* see inside anyone's head. Then I try to suggest that after revealing their hidden fears, they may well discover that these fears are not unique. Their apprehensions are shared by many people; once they have admitted to them, they should begin to experience a sense of relief.

Other people, anticipating that their therapist will not believe them, rely principally on their own interpretation of what is true. Worse, after a person has made a shameful or secretive disclosure, they fear the therapist will respond badly: that is, either laugh or be outraged, angry, or indifferent.

As real as these fears may be, I find that good psychiatrists or therapists will always be accepting and compassionate. Part of their trustworthiness rests in their being receptive—responding honestly and directly. It is important for people to understand that many, if not most, therapists have undergone therapy themselves. The therapist's own experience of fears of disclosure is often the source of considerable insight and empathy. They understand what it is like being on the other side of the couch.

Finally, I find many people fear that psychiatrists may not discover the real cause of their symptoms. They dread the idea that their psychiatric treatment will take many years and still be inconclusive. Although it is certainly possible that treatment may be protracted, this is unusual. The vast number of psychiatric symptoms or problems, such as specific types of depression and anxiety, are time-limited. Unless they become exaggerated, most of them disappear within a given, sometimes predictable, period of time—usually about three to six months.

Resistance to Psychiatric Drugs

I believe that many people share a deeply felt ambivalence toward taking psychiatric medication, even when they are admittedly sick and their doctor recommends drugs as part of their treatment.

When people become physically ill, most of them expect to get well and believe that the medicine their doctor prescribes will play a role in their eventual recovery. Many will even *expect* medication and are disappointed if they don't receive any. But when it comes to psychiatric illnesses, this pattern of care that routinely includes medication differs. Unless their symptoms have been severe and disruptive, I find that most people initially resist the idea of psychiatric drug use, even if it is recommended as part of their treatment.

This resistance is very understandable since most of us share a bedrock aversion toward anything that may substantially alter the way we feel about ourselves—especially in a way we cannot control. People fear that taking a psychiatric drug will adversely affect their brain, the very organ that controls their consciousness and, in some way, affects their individuality. Psychiatric drugs can change that which is unseen, poorly understood, and probably malfunctioning. This power strikes them more as mystery than science.

A related problem is the identification of the person with the disease or disorder: "I am a depressed person" instead of "I am suffering from depression." As a result, these people see the drug as treating them and not the disorder.

It is important for people to appreciate the fact that drugs are not designed to wrest control from anyone. On the contrary, if they are used sensibly and under proper supervision, drugs can restore order and stability to the lives of millions of people who are unable, usually temporarily, to function under normal circumstances.

A typical case of someone who initially resisted medication is a forty-five-year-old man who, after two months of psychiatric counseling, was sent to me for psychiatric assessment. I diagnosed his problem as depression and recommended an antidepressant as part of his treatment program.

He initially confessed to feeling a little ashamed that he was depressed. He viewed depression as less acceptable than certain other diagnoses, such as anxiety. Worse yet, he did not like the idea of taking medication to control the "inner workings of his feeling life."

During the first two weeks of therapy, he resented taking the drug; it was, in his words, a daily reminder of his "sense of failure." He viewed it as a public acknowledgment of something he did not want to disclose to others. He also wanted to be reassured that he would not have to take the drug for the rest of his life. I told him that there was no indication that he would have to do so. He seemed comforted when I told him that probably less than 1 percent of all people taking psychiatric drugs *must* take them for a period of several years.

He eventually accepted the necessity for the medication, and when we changed the medication to a one-a-day dose, he was able to take the drug at night in complete privacy.

One final note: this person needed to take the medication for less than five months and today, years later, remains free of any depressive symptoms.

Now I am going to contradict myself. I believe that we are in the midst of a significant change in attitudes toward psychiatric medications. For example, we doctors wrote more than 1,600,000,000 prescriptions in 1988 (the actual number of pills is probably greater than 100 billion). The lion's share of these drugs, antibiotics, represented six of the top ten drugs. But ranking third among all drugs prescribed that year was XANAX, a tranquilizer. Two of the best-selling new drugs on the market are HALCION, used to treat insomnia, and PROZAC, an antidepressant. And the sales of psychiatric drugs overall are growing. While many people still have deep reservations about the use of psychiatric drugs, millions of other Americans have developed a gradual acceptance—if not overreliance—on them.

Millions of people have come to see minor tranquilizers as an answer to the stress and tension of their everyday lives. This is unfortunate. There is nothing wrong with feeling sad, depressed, or discouraged. It's probably healthy; the world itself is often sad, depressing, and discouraging. What is not healthy, however, is the use of drugs to avoid those common feelings altogether, especially outside of a psychiatric or therapeutic context.

A quite legitimate concern explicitly associated with psychiatric medications is drug dependence. I frequently reassure people that the drug they take will not create some irreversible change in them; once they start taking the drug, they will not inevitably become chemically or emotionally dependent on it. Drug dependency is always possible, but never likely, especially if you follow your physician's instructions. And if such a condition develops, a physician can usually ease you off the drug without any serious problems.

People also ask me whether their symptoms will return: "Will I get sicker if I stop taking the drug?" This is unlikely if they follow their physician's instructions.

The good news is that, over time, most psychiatric medications work to the benefit of the person taking the drug. If the medication regimen prescribed by a psychiatrist is followed correctly, most people will not have any serious trouble with the drug or its effects. Identifying the correct drug and establishing appropriate dosage levels may require some adjustments—like switching to other drugs within the same family. But most people are able to take psychiatric medication as a safe and effective part of their recovery and healing.

Compliance and Drug Use

The success of any treatment is dependent upon your faithfully taking the required dosage at the time agreed upon. It is widely accepted, however, that as many as 30 percent of all people taking psychiatric medication under a doctor's supervision fail to fully recover or suffer a relapse in their treatment because of improper use of their medication. Consequently, you and your psychiatrist should work out a drug schedule that is simple and unobtrusive enough to make it easy for you to remember when to take your drugs and that does not cause undue public attention to your treatment.

The reasons for noncompliance range from the trivial to the serious, from the seemingly rational to the highly irrational. For example, some people will stop taking their medications because they are angry at someone else or the schedule has become too difficult to follow. Other people quit because they think the drug is not doing any good or they can no longer tolerate the "defect" in their behavior. Still others stop out of a fear that they will become addicted to the drug. I have had patients skip their medications because it interfered with important social rituals such as evening cocktails, given the prohibition over the use of alcohol. Another factor contributing to not taking medication is the inability to open the container. Although admirably childproof, some container tops may also be adult-proof for elderly, arthritic, or debilitated adults. Rather than face embarrassment many adults will simply not take the medication. Transferring to a simpler operating container is a ready solution. With the cost of new medications climbing, many people cannot afford their drugs. Unwilling to tell their therapist, patients often do without and suffer in silence. However, older medications that are equally effective have inexpensive generic forms. It is important to ask about these medications and take advantage of their lower prices. For that matter, if you have any concerns about your medications, share them with your physician.

The most common early complaint, once patients begin their medications, is that their medicine doesn't work. Usually the discontent is premature since they have not taken the medicine for a sufficient period of time for it to be effective (most drugs require at least a week, some many weeks, before clinical benefits become evident). The drug may also not be effective because its dosage is not correct. In these instances, anxious patients often need to be reminded that their medications may require one or more dosage adjustments before an appropriate level can be established.

Another early complaint concerns anticipated side effects. Again, these concerns are often premature since many side effects become less troublesome or even vanish over time. However, if the symptoms were to persist, it may be a reason to either adjust the dosage or prescribe a different medication altogether.

I have found that anxiety can produce exaggerated expectations. Anxious or highly distressed patients often want a rapid, almost magical, relief from or cure of their affliction. While understandable, such an attitude can undermine a successful experience with the medication. It is necessary that your physician explain, among other things, the process of the drug therapy and the time frame and sequence of likely changes that you may experience with the medication. Not only should your doctor entertain any questions you have but he should actively elicit from you any doubts, anecdotal prejudices, or fears you may have regarding the medication. This process builds the needed quality of empathy and trust you want in your relationship with your doctor. And even if you will not be seeing your doctor on a regular basis, you need to confidently know and anticipate something of the experience you may have with your medications.

On the other hand, if you feel unable to speak candidly about your experience with your medications, we often see something called the "iceberg effect." This is a situation in which patients keep issues hidden they believe are important but cannot risk revealing. Common examples are sexual difficulties or incontinence and unvoiced doubts about the need for the medication or fears that it will never be effective. If their concerns remain undiscussed and untreated, patients frequently will resolve their anxiety by either prematurely stopping the drug or using it in ways that render the drug ineffective.

It is almost self-evident that people who accept and understand the appropriateness of their therapy, and especially the justification for their medications, increase the likelihood of their having a successful outcome. Conversely, I have seen in my own practice numerous instances in which someone's negative attitude toward his or her medication subtly undermined or diminished its effectiveness. My point is that your belief is linked to your behavior. People who have no obvious problems of memory or confusion, but who harbor unexpressed or unresolved fears about their medication, frequently find it difficult to remember to take their medications on time, or will consistently forget about the middle dose of a multiple-dose regimen. If they bring this to my attention, I will often inquire into whether they have any conflicted feelings about the need for their drug regimen. What I most often learn is that they feared they might become addicted to the drug and, thus, consciously or unconsciously attempted to maintain a modest dose. Yet, when reassured that their fears were unfounded and the patient made upward adjustments in their dosage, their symptoms decreased. Again, many psychiatric conditions will not improve without the benefit of medication, and others frankly get much worse if medication is delayed or improperly taken.

Noncompliance is usually more prevalent among people who take medication over extended periods of time, especially to prevent or decrease the recurrence of an episode. In conventional medicines, for example, noncompliance frequently occurs among those treated for hypertension and diabetes—two diseases that require long-term or lifelong use of medicines. Among psychiatric medications, people treated with LITHIUM for manic depressive illness often digress from their doctor's very specific instructions regarding their medication as do people who require long-term use of low-dose neuroleptic drugs for the treatment of schizophrenia or delusional disorders.

Once these long-term or maintenance programs have eliminated symptoms for a few months, some people are apt to stop their medication without notifying their doctor. Essentially, they believe that the medication is no longer needed—they no longer have symptoms—that they have been cured of the underlying problem. Unfortunately, not only is this unwise, but unsafe. Only their doctor is trained to determine whether the treatment should be changed or halted. The very lack of symptoms could be the primary reason for continuing the drug regimen rather than discontinuing it.

For people on maintenance medication, I like to institute drug holidays, that is, regular days or weekends that are drug free. I find that this practice provides a break from the sometimes mechanizing routine of the drug schedule and reduces the incidence of noncompliance. These drug holidays can also be helpful for patients who experience diminished sexual desire or performance. Many psychiatric conditions, such as depression, which may lead to lack of sexual desire, are often wrongly attributed to the medication. Medications can and do, however, interfere with sexual function. Unfortunately, these side effects often go unreported.

No single strategy has been able to overcome this difficulty other than the long-suffering patience of the partner. However, various medications such as yohimbine, the antihistamine PERIACTIN, or the Parkinson's disease medication bromocriptine may give some relief, though they're not consistent. The worst offenders, and now most commonly used offenders, are SSRI antidepressants, such as PROZAC, ZOLOFT, and PAXIL. I have found that stopping the medication over the weekend may arrest the sexual problem; many patients have reported that a break in the routine has done away with their anorgasmia, or failure to achieve an orgasm, probably the most common of drug-related sexual problems.

If you find that you are resenting your medication, talk to your doctor about possible changes. Resentment can lead to inattentiveness and, eventually, willful misuse of the drug. Do not make any upward or downward adjustments in your dosages or schedule without your doctor's knowledge and permission. Most important, tell your doctor if you want or intend to stop the medication. If unsupervised, it may not only delay long-term therapeutic goals but it may produce a full return of all symptoms. (For more information on the importance of following a prescribed drug schedule, see "Misconceptions That Lead to Misuse," page 78).

Medication Schedules

Different drugs require or allow for different dosage schedules. An antidepressant such as PROZAC (page 119) can be given as a single and fixed regulated dose. (A convenience of a single-dose medication like PROZAC is that it allows for the drug to be taken in the morning.) Other medications, such as those antianxiety drugs that have no *latency* period, can be taken as needed. They work immediately, and a single dose can be taken only when symptoms appear.

Most psychiatric medications, however, begin with divided doses, which means the doses are taken at various times of the day. Once a steady-state blood level is established through the administration of divided doses, then a single dose may be used to maintain the proper level. To simplify a divided-dose schedule to a single-dose regimen is really worthwhile, as there may be no better strategy for ensuring drug compliance.

Different psychiatric illnesses also require different treatment schedules. At the very outset of therapy, your doctor may tell you that the drug will be prescribed for only three months. Certain types of depression naturally last about this long. Establishing a certain finite period of time for drug use can also be viewed as an expression of your doctor's confidence that, with the help of the medication, your symptoms will cease by that time. I also believe that, whenever appropriate, announcing to the patient that the drug will be used for only a limited time is helpful because it underscores the relative role of the medication in the therapeutic process: namely, drugs are usually not a permanent part of someone's therapy.

However, for many of the biologically based illnesses, fixed-time regimens are unrealistic. If your problem were manic-depression, for example, the planned drug therapy would probably be for an indeterminate period of time since the course of these illnesses can be chronic and recurrent.

In summary, if you are prescribed a psychiatric drug, it will probably be for a fixed period of time. If, however, your doctor cannot tell you in advance how long you will have to take the drug, do not panic. Your rate of recovery will determine how much medication you will take and how long.

Proper Role of Medications

Psychiatric drugs are designed to diminish or eliminate unwanted symptoms. If successful, the drug will cause the symptoms to disappear. However, if the drug only *diminishes* your symptoms, you should not consider it a failure. In the broader context of the therapy, it is a step toward full elimination of the symptoms. Further success may require, in some cases, the help of other medications. It is only through trial and error that we sometimes learn which is the best drug for someone. But, once we identify the correct drug or drugs, psychiatric drugs are generally able to suppress or eliminate most or all the common psychological symptoms.

Another role of psychiatric drugs is the prevention of cyclical disorders—illnesses that come and go, sometimes in a recognizable pattern. Two examples are LITHIUM, a maintenance medication used in the prevention of manic-depressive illness, and DILANTIN, prescribed to prevent grand mal seizures.

Another point worth mentioning is that psychiatric drugs should not be used to improve levels of functioning beyond what people are used to or what is considered normal for them. These drugs are restorative in that they are meant to return someone to former levels of functioning, namely, over the impaired levels they experienced before taking the medicine. In this regard, I am reminded of the joke about the patient who, following his operation, asked his surgeon if he could play the piano. When the surgeon said, "Yes, of course," the patient seemed puzzled, and replied, "That's odd, because I've never played the piano before."

In the larger picture of rehabilitation, psychiatric drugs are only tools. They are facilitators; they are not the total solution. It is important to understand this limited role of drugs. Believing a drug does it all is to hand over your autonomy when you are always the responsible agent for change. As I mentioned earlier, psychiatric drugs are intended to treat your problem and not you.

Finding the Right Drug

Psychiatric drugs do not produce uniform results. Side effects and recovery rates differ from patient to patient. We all have unique central nervous systems and metabolic systems: we react differently to various stimuli and absorb foods or drugs at different levels of efficiency. Consequently, no *one* medication is effective in all people, or effective in the same fashion. Because of this unpredictability, the process of finding the correct psychiatric drug is often governed by trial and error. It often means upward or downward adjustments in dosage, or switching to other medications before the correct (or best) drug and dosage are found.

For a variety of reasons, people may resist the intended action of their medication; they unconsciously struggle against getting better. One example would be those people who have made a psychic investment in their illness. I have treated some people who converted their illness into an asset, though it is largely an unconscious process. They came to accept their illness—especially one that has been officially sanctioned by a psychiatric treatment—as a permit to regress to a dependent state. They used their treatment as a request for more attention and expressions of love from their family members. Or they sought, through their illness, to avoid responsibilities, such as work or family obligations. And the principal verification of their need for exceptional care and concern was the psychiatric medication.

These people frustrated their treatment by developing a psychological dependency on the illness, however unconsciously. Making the drug both ineffective and necessary, they developed an implicit drug dependency. In these rare circumstances, there may be no medicine that would be effective. And it is always a sad situation: neither the drug nor the doctor can help because these people cannot or will not help themselves. Oddly enough, this is further evidence that control often remains more in the hands of the individual than in the drug or the therapist.

Some readers may want to know if there are guidelines by which they could measure the effectiveness of their drug. For example, how much time should be allowed before an ineffective drug should be switched? Frankly, drug effectiveness is a matter that should be discussed with your doctor. If you see someone on a regular basis—this is called *continuity of treatment*—you do not need specific guidelines. In all likelihood, your doctor will tell you which cluster of symptoms should be treated and, perhaps, when you might expect relief from them. In any event, any and all progress is something that you should routinely discuss with your doctor.

In Chapter 6, where I profile all the most commonly used psychiatric drugs, I list under the "Course of Treatment" the likely stages of the drug's effectiveness, which may be of some help. In addition, if for some reason your drug remains ineffective after six weeks, I would say that it is time to review the drug and the medication schedule with your doctor.

People Authorized to Prescribe Psychiatric Medications

People obtain psychiatric medication from many sources—some authorized, others not. Among those sources licensed to dispense psychiatric medications are medical doctors or primary care physicians, such as internists, pediatricians, and gynecologists. This list also includes dentists.

Though these medical professionals have no specific training in psychiatric medications, they are licensed to prescribe psychiatric drugs for specific conditions, such as preparation for a colonoscopy, dental procedures, or biopsies. In such instances, where a relaxed patient is vital for the procedure to be successful, a minor tranquilizer can be useful. However, the medication should be given on an ad hoc basis and its use should be restricted only to that specific occasion of anxiety.

Situations in which psychiatric drugs are prescribed by medical doctors vary. For example, I know of many people who have received a prescription for a tranquilizer to treat their performance anxiety. Also, I know that some doctors have prescribed an anti-depressant to a patient they know well and who has displayed symptoms of depression for months. I am opposed to this practice, at least in principle, because the primary care physician is not only less qualified to give medication on an extended basis than a licensed psychiatrist, but they are usually not trained to monitor the psychiatric symptoms for which the drug was prescribed.

If professional restrictions are not well observed, that is, when someone is given an open-ended prescription for a tranquilizer, a genuine occasion for drug abuse develops. Over the past fifteen years, I have seen emergency rooms receive more and more people who have overdosed on a minor tranquilizer. Ten years ago, the drug was VALIUM (page 250), but there has been a progressive decrease in the amount of VALIUM prescribed since then. Now, I see more ATIVAN (page 263) and XANAX (page 261) as abused drugs. However, without regard to the specific tranquilizer involved, what we learned at Bellevue was that these people often had been given large amounts of, or an open-ended prescription for, the drug by their primary care physician for nonspecific symptoms, such as tension or stress.

No patient should have de facto unlimited access to a psychiatric drug. A prescription for as many as one hundred pills at a time with multiple refills permits unsupervised use of a seductive and addicting drug. Prescribing drugs in these quantities not only discourages people from seeing a physician, it makes it quite unnecessary. Whether done intentionally or not, these are the kinds of actions that promote drug misuse.

The second group of individuals who prescribe psychiatric medications is made up of general psychiatrists, that is, doctors trained in adult psychiatry who treat a whole spectrum of adult disorders. These "general practitioners" of psychiatry are reasonably well-versed in a variety of psychotherapies and, of course, psychiatric medications. Moreover, their postgraduate education includes training in medicine and neurology; this enables them to distinguish between a neurological and a psychiatric problem. For example, certain types of seizures—a neurological or a medical problem—can cause someone to suffer from a serious personality dissociation. That is, someone suffering from a seizure might leave home or their office on impulse and have no memory of it when they recover from the seizure hours later. Such a problem would have to be treated by a neurologist and not a psychiatrist. However, to some health-care professionals, these symptoms might appear to be solely psychiatric.

A third group is psychopharmacologists, whom patients see either in private practice or in clinics. These people are specialists in psychiatric medicine, but their view of treatment often remains rather narrow and restrictive. Their expertise lies primarily with the *drug* and not the *patient*: their focus is on the efficacy of the drug and making appropriate judgments about its specific action and the likelihood of adverse reactions.

Other therapists include psychologists, psychiatric social workers, psychiatric nurses, and the clergy. These people are not allowed to prescribe medicine, but they can refer patients to licensed physicians. For example, psychiatric nurses, who usually work in clinics or hospitals, are directly supervised by a licensed physician, psychiatrist, or psychopharmacologist. In addition to referring you to a psychiatrist or someone authorized to prescribe medication, health-care professionals in this group may also offer an opinion about which drug should be prescribed. However, talking about a specific drug at this juncture should be considered premature at best since a specific psychiatric drug is usually selected only after a complete psychiatric diagnosis.

Why Psychiatric Medications Are Prescribed

The therapeutic purposes for which a drug is prescribed are called *indications*. The indications for psychiatric medications are generally quite specific. For example, the drug INDERAL (page 266) is commonly prescribed for performance anxiety on an as-needed basis. However, INDERAL would be totally ineffective for a chronic state of anxiety, otherwise called a *generalized anxiety disorder*.

All psychiatric symptoms are potential clues that can lead to a larger context, which may in turn explain the reasons for those symptoms. Psychiatric drugs should never be prescribed for symptoms outside this therapeutic context—not even for something as seemingly common as insomnia. It's not good medicine. The first step, then, should be a thorough psychiatric diagnosis conducted by a psychiatrist. The diagnosis may reveal that a single symptom, such as insomnia or anxiety, may be the result solely of a specific event or circumstance, such as the loss of a job or a troubled relationship. Then, again, it may be related to another larger problem.

A standard analogy is a fever, a symptom that is often linked to an underlying illness. Now, if a mild fever abates shortly after you take aspirin, and does not return, you may rightly consider it unrelated to any other illness and have no further interest in it. But if a fever has persisted for more than a day, changed in its intensity, and/or has resisted usual treatment, it is likely that it is associated with a more serious ailment or infection.

The same is true of psychiatric symptoms. If your insomnia or anxiety were accompanied by symptoms of listlessness or social withdrawal, your therapist might have cause to believe that an underlying problem exists—such as a depressive illness. In such a situation, the treatment for the insomnia or anxiety, including the choice of drug, would include a diagnosis and treatment of the underlying depression as well.

In summary, *psychiatric medications should not be prescribed except following a diagnosis of the patient.* It trivializes the proper role of these drugs to believe they are used for symptom relief alone. In some circumstances, it is clinically dangerous to medicate without a proper diagnosis.

Certain symptoms of such profundity or seriousness call for psychiatric medication even before the evaluation process is completed. Typical examples are a wish to hurt yourself (associated with feelings of hopelessness); a wish to die (so to end the pain of separation); a belief that you are being followed, spied upon, or controlled by other people; or a belief you are hearing or seeing things that others do not see and for which there is no consensual validation. Additional behaviors that might warrant psychiatric medication before a complete diagnosis is available would be those indicative of profound eating disorders: excessive fasting, gross and uncontrolled eating binges, or excessive use of diuretics or cathartics. But in most instances, a psychiatric evaluation is recommended before someone begins taking psychiatric drugs.

What Your Doctor Needs to Know

Personal Health

As I mentioned in the previous section, before I prescribe a psychiatric medication for my patients, I make a complete evaluation— not only of their psychiatric needs but their health history as well. I especially need to know if they are suffering from a physical illness or specific allergy. Without this information, I might prescribe a drug that could possibly provoke or aggravate a current illness or trigger an allergic reaction. In some instances, an incorrectly prescribed drug can be life-threatening.

I can recall an instance in which a thirty-four-year-old woman was given monoamine-oxidase (MAO) inhibitor, a powerful antidepressant drug, in her treatment for depression. Unknown to her doctor, the woman had also been taking, intermittently, some cold medicine she had bought in her local drugstore the previous year. Because she believed the nonprescription medication was unimportant, she never told her doctor about it. This was regrettable in that the medication contained pressor agents (chemicals that elevate blood pressure), such as phenylpropalamine. As a result, within a week she was complaining of severe headaches and a bloody nose. Her problem was that she was suffering from dangerously high blood pressure, or hypertension. As soon as she stopped taking the cold medicine, however, the symptoms stopped.

Another equally important medical problem that affects psychiatric medication is the problem of seizures. Certain medications, such as antidepressants, may induce a convulsive episode in someone who is susceptible. And it is not unheard of for people who did not tell their doctor about their early history of heart disease to experience altered heart rhythms and some anxious moments after receiving an antidepressant.

In all these instances, the individual usually has failed to tell the doctor something important about their health status, or the doctor has failed to ask.

Needless to say, it is essential to let your doctor know of any psychiatric medications you have taken. In addition, I always want to learn what kind of attitude or feelings someone holds toward a previous drug experience. If a drug worked in the past, it should receive first consideration—that is, if the circumstances making the drug necessary are similar. In addition to a personal history of drug use, I want to know if there is a family history with any psychiatric drug. It can be helpful to know how a member of your family has responded to a particular drug, especially if he or she suffered from the same condition as yours. Drug histories suggest that, given similar circumstances, a drug that has failed or worked for one member of the family at some time may behave in a corresponding manner for another.

In addition, family histories are important because certain psychiatric illnesses are hereditary: that is, families share a susceptibility or risk of them. A few years ago, I treated a grandmother for agoraphobia, which is a fear of open spaces. Then two years after the onset of her treatment, I began to treat the daughter for the same phobia. In both instances, I was able to use the same medication successfully. Ironically enough, there was evidence that the son, of the third generation, also had a similar phobic illness which was developing at the time. This five-year-old intensely feared going to school; he had *school phobia*. He was experiencing a form of separation anxiety that was related to his mother's and grandmother's agoraphobia, which manifested itself as a fear of not being able to leave their own house.

Drug Interactions

During your first, or at least subsequent, visit with your psychiatrist, it is important that you tell the doctor about any medications you are taking, *including over-the-counter medications*. This discussion should include any changes or additions to your medication schedule which may influence the effectiveness of the drug(s) you will be taking. You need to avoid taking two or more drugs that work on the same central nervous system in your body. The combined effects could produce highly exaggerated effects—far more than you or your doctor want.

You might think that it is unlikely that you would forget to tell your doctor about another drug you were taking, especially one that would cause such a serious problem. However, this happens far more often than you might believe. When asked by their psychiatrists if they are taking any medications, many people fail to mention nonprescription medicines, since—as someone once told me—"they're not real medicines."

I find that many elderly patients fail to tell their psychiatrist or therapist that they take diuretics, probably because they have been taking them for several years and simply forget. In one instance, such an omission had serious consequences. A sixty-eight-year-old woman was given LITHIUM by her psychiatrist. She was also taking a diuretic, apparently for several years. Within a few days she began to complain of confusion, facial twitching, and disorientation. The action of the diuretic was causing a salt imbalance; abnormally high levels of LITHIUM developed in her body. In effect, she was being poisoned by the LITHIUM. When the doctor questioned her more closely about the use of any other drugs, she realized that she had forgotten to tell him about her diuretics. The symptoms disappeared as soon as she was taken off both drugs.

A second example: two drugs that have the same action. Someone taking ALDOMET, which is a drug for the treatment of hypertension, should not take a neuroleptic tranquilizer such as THORAZINE, since the two drugs—the antihypertensive and the tranquilizer—would both act to lower blood pressure. The result would be a significant, perhaps dangerous, decrease in standing blood pressure.

Another example of two drugs that both act as central nervous system (CNS) depressants: alcohol and THORAZINE. When taken together, these two drugs can be powerfully sedating and dependent-forming. If active alcoholics take a hypnotic sedative like VALIUM to calm their alcohol-related anxiety symptoms, they can become very sick. If unchecked or in sufficient quantities, these types of drug combinations can produce severe central nervous system depression. They can also be deadly.

The pain reliever DEMEROL and monoamine-oxidase (MAO) inhibitors together can be equally fatal. One such case involved the daughter of a prominent New York journalist. It seems that her physician did not know that she had been given MAO inhibitor by her psychiatrist. As a result, the DEMEROL she received caused her death.

Another drug-interaction problem involves a drug that *heightens* the effects of other drugs. By slowing down the metabolism of a psychiatric medication, another drug can actually prolong or increase its effect. An example is (1) DEPAKENE (page 282), a drug for people who have wide and rapid mood changes, and (2) an antidepressant. When taken together, the DEPAKENE can increase the potency of the antidepressant beyond what is desired because it inhibits metabolism, both its own and that of others. The net result is that more of both drugs stay in the body longer. In such a situation, your doctor would monitor your blood levels and probably reduce the dose of one or both drugs.

An opposite situation exists when a drug *diminishes* the effectiveness of another psychiatric drug. For example, TEGRETOL (page 280) accelerates the breakdown of other drugs. As a result, if you take TEGRETOL with another medication, it will hasten the breakdown of the other drug, reduce the amount available to your body and, in effect, reduce its overall effectiveness. So whenever taking TEGRETOL, it is necessary to monitor blood levels frequently and, perhaps, upwardly adjust the dosage of the medication, or adjust the dosage of the other drug that is given with it.

A fourth category of potential drug interactions occurs when one drug *cancels* the effects of another drug because it has the opposite action on the same system. Often these drug interactions cannot be fully anticipated. An example would be the case of a sixty-two-year-old man who was being treated with SYMMETREL (page 232) for his Parkinson's disease. But because he was highly agitated, he was also given a sedative in the form of THORAZINE to quiet him. Although the tranquilizer was not *contraindicated*, which is to say it was not inappropriate to prescribe, the interaction between the two drugs unexpectedly made him more agitated. The reason is this: SYMMETREL, the drug he was taking for his Parkinsonism, increases the availability of dopamine to the brain. On the other hand, the action of the tranquilizer THORAZINE blocks dopamine. So, instead of working together, as they certainly could have—one drug reducing the tremors and the other the agitation—they produced opposite effects.

As you can see, drug interactions are not necessarily the result of intentional misuse or an inappropriate prescription. As in the case of SINEMET and THORAZINE, although there is a potential risk of a drug interaction, they can be used concurrently in many cases with success. In other instances, however, when two or more drugs pose a clear risk of an adverse reaction, they are contraindicated, that is, they should definitely not be taken together. Such an instance would be the potentially lethal combination of alcohol and tranquilizers mentioned earlier.

The circumstances that most often lead to unwanted drug interactions are those involving ignorance: taking a drug without knowing or realizing that the presence of another could produce a severe adverse reaction. This is why it is so important to tell your doctor about *all* the drugs you are currently taking, as well as those you have recently taken. Some medications require a *washout* period before another drug can be used: that is, a period of drug abstinence is required before another drug can be taken. (See "Washout Period," page 86.) So, normally very safe drugs can become quite unsafe in combination.

At this point, I want to emphasize that the practice of self-diagnosing is always bad medicine. Nevertheless, some people tend to create their own drug-treatment regimens based on their own diagnosis. My objection is not that a certain drug combination may be inappropriate; it is based solely on the fact that psychiatric drug treatments should *always* be supervised by a psychiatrist. There are *always* possible responses or drug reactions that you are not trained to handle.

For example, if people have trouble getting to sleep while taking the antidepressant PROZAC, they might decide to take HALCION, especially if it had been a combination their doctor had prescribed in the past. In their confidence, they decide to prescribe the same combination for themselves.

Now, the danger of playing doctor and creating one's own program of self-medication is that it involves uninformed risk. Someone taking both PROZAC and HALCION may develop a day-time anxiety if he abruptly stops taking the HALCION (anxiety is a very likely symptom, I might add, especially if taken for several months). To treat the anxiety, this person might start taking the antianxiety drug XANAX, but without allowing for the washout period needed for HALCION. This is a perfect setup for a number of potential adverse reactions.

My point is that a supervising physician would not allow these situations to develop. The use of psychiatric medications always involves some risk, however small, for which you want a trained professional at your side.

Prozac Phenomena

Perhaps no other drug in recent history has been as heralded or vilified as PROZAC. Promoted by the media and personal testimony, this new antidepressant was received as a miracle drug that would change people's lives and their fortunes. It has been vilified in turn by various nonconventional self-help groups as a drug that promotes violent or suicidal thoughts and behavior. Both claims are blatantly false.

It is not fully clear how PROZAC earned its exaggerated reputation. PROZAC is a very effective antidepressant that has helped many people with quite legitimate clinical problems, and several celebrities publicly and enthusiastically endorsed the drug after they experienced welcome relief from their own symptoms. One likely explanation for their rhapsodic claims of euphoria is that the drug supposedly provided them with a feeling of blessed relief. Patients claimed that it magically changed them, once the depressive and imprisoning symptoms of their disease lifted. Other antidepressive medications have provided many patients the same relief, too, but probably not with as few side effects or with the same rate of success.

In the midst of its harvest of praise, PROZAC has also received harsh press from groups who saw the drug's "transformative powers" as a threat to their existence. One self-help group attacked the drug as a control agent designed to undermine the authority of its members by controlling their minds. Others felt that talk therapy would be co-opted by the simple dispensing of this medication. A case in point is the Washington psychologist who immediately referred most, if not all, of his patients to a physician in order to be placed on PROZAC. He is facing charges of malpractice by his state board. And in one science magazine, the drug was heralded, though admittedly as an intentional hyperbole, as the "death of therapy." It could be argued, as some commentators have, that the wholesale embrace of PROZAC is part of a broader effort in our society to medicate the ordinary. People have too often viewed their everyday angst as clinical depression that required medication, and, in many instances, the drug of choice was PROZAC.

On the other hand, the press had also reported claims that the drug was dangerous since it produced suicidal episodes in some patients. Again, these claims are unfounded. Except in those instances of a patient who is predisposed to such behavior, or has received an overdose, the general side effects of PROZAC do not include such dire consequences. And if any disconcerting side effects should occur with PROZAC, they are relatively short lasting.

Unfortunately, more than a few patients in my practice have refused, at least initially, to take PROZAC since they were frightened by the adverse and irresponsible publicity surrounding the drug. But others were also put off because of its exaggerated favorable reputation. They were frightened by what they saw as an extravagantly powerful life-changing drug that would assume control over their lives. Some thought it would even lead to an inevitable addiction.

Some people are afraid to stop taking the drug once it successfully diminishes or eliminates their symptoms, they so believe the positive changes are solely the work of the medication. If they were to discontinue the drug, they believe, they would regress to their former misery. This is an understandable fear given the power some people give over to the drug, but I don't recall my patients expressing such faith and fear in other antidepressive medications that had also produced favorable outcomes. For those patients who fear terminating PROZAC, I remind them that talk therapy or psychology can usually consolidate the affective and attitudinal changes that have occurred in them while taking the drug, a point often missed by some primary-care physicians who have given out antidepressants to their patients with disappointing results. In those instances, I suspect that the physician and the patient both have assumed that, like an antibiotic, the medication would work silently and passively. The fact of the matter is that the role of these drugs is to support the patient's recovery, and while they may provide some temporary relief of symptoms, they cannot be said to cure the problem. The activity of the medication is to make therapy more successful by freeing up the patient's energy, where they become less self-absorbed and better able to interact with their therapist.

Yes, symptoms may return if the drug is discontinued prematurely. It may also lose its faulted power on its own due to the "poop out" phenomenon. All this means is that, over time, the drug often will lose some or all of its original effectiveness for many patients.

The hoopla over PROZAC, however, did promote the current research exploration of the neurotransmitter serotonin. As a result, four of the newest antidepressants on the market affect serotonin transmission. Serotonin was not a new discovery of the developers of PROZAC. The role of serotonin has been known since earlier generations of antidepressants, which affected serotonin along with the norepinephrine systems. But the advent of SSRIs drew greater attention to the function of the serotonin receptor because, while we don't really know everywhere the drug actually goes in the nervous system, these drugs act overwhelmingly on this one. In PROZAC we have a drug that was "cleaner" than the others in that it appeared to act even more selectively on the serotonin receptor alone. For the patient this means fewer side effects and perhaps greater efficacy.

The pharmaceutical business is often market driven. The commercial success of PROZAC sponsored an intense interest in developing clones of the drug. As a result of this serotonin research, we learned a great more about the serotonin system on which PROZAC works. For example, new research revealed the existence of at least seven distinct types of serotonin receptor—namely, all serotonin receptors were not the same. Because researchers had identified these different types of serotonin cells, they could create drugs, such as the four newest antidepressive drugs on the market, EFFEXOR, ZOLOFT, PAXIL, and SERZONE. Since these drugs are selective of a particular type of serotonin receptor, they can separate the different depressive, anxiety-ridden, migraine-producing, and emetic (vomiting) effects of serotonin.

A second major breakthrough has been the discovery of the role of serotonin in psychotic illness. Researchers believe that the neurotransmitter serotonin may play a role in overcoming the negative symptoms of psychosis that had been resistant to drug treatment, such as the lack of initiative and spontaneity, or the flat or blunted feelings of many patients. These discoveries have been incorporated in the new atypical antipsychotic drug, RISPERIDOL.

Two treatment-emergent symptoms, symptoms that occur after more than a week of drug use, have been reported with SSRIs. One is the sudden loss of drug effect known as "poop out," where the drug will lose its effectiveness over time, though when this may occur varies from patient to patient. The other symptom is patient poop out, since many people experience the onset of fatigue six to eight hours after taking the drug. Although speculative, both effects are thought to be due to excessive serotonin and decreased nerve sensitivity. One strategy, referred to as a drug holiday, is to stop the medicine for two weeks, which temporarily reduces the level of serotonin and permits the nerve to recharge the system. The other strategy takes an opposite view. It raises the dosage of medication to increase the level of the neurotransmitter and overcome the assumed temporary blockade. In my experience, the latter strategy runs the risk of drowning the receptor.

TWO

How Psychiatric Drugs Work in the Body

The Central Nervous System

At this point, to broaden what will still be a very general description of how psychiatric drugs work, I first want to talk briefly about the principal components of the central nervous system (CNS).

The CNS is a complex two-way wiring system over which the brain communicates and exercises central control of our body. The system monitors events in the periphery of the body—from the tips of the fingers and large organs of the gut to the perceptual system (e.g., the eyes and ears)—and relays the information back to the brain. There it integrates and interprets the information and responds. By controlling the system centrally and feeding back peripherally, the brain constantly monitors both what goes on inside our body and our body's relationship to the external world.

Since every pain, every change in position, every stimulus in the body is sensed and transmitted centrally to the brain, the brain and nervous system function together as the central control for our body. In other words, the brain and the body are not two distinct systems. Therefore, not only are all sensations and events occur-

28

ring in the body recorded in the brain, but through this two-way feedback system, events going on in the brain—e.g., anxiety, depression, or stress in general—affect all the organs of the body.

Principal Units of the CNS

The central nervous system is made up of a series of functional units—the largest being the brain, the spinal cord, and the brainstem—that carry out complex and separate tasks. In the brain, some of the functional units are anatomically discrete or have a very specific location, such as the motor system for speech. Other functional units, although anatomically linked, are scattered throughout the brain. One is the limbic system, an area of the brain associated with anxiety; it crosses a number of anatomical areas.

The exterior of the brain is protected by an outer shell or skull (skull means *bowl*) made of bone. Inside this skull, additional protection is provided by a series of membranes that surround the brain—the *blood brain barrier*. This barrier selectively and actively admits certain substances circulating throughout the blood system of the body. Those substances seen as hostile to the delicate nerve cells of the brain are rejected. Such rejected substances are said to be unable to "cross the blood brain barrier."

From the brain the central nervous system extends through the spinal cord—also encased in bone for protection—and out to a series of peripheral nerves and ganglia that extend throughout the body. What connects your brain to your spinal cord is your brainstem. It controls many of your vital functions, such as breathing, blood circulation, and balance. The purpose of the peripheral nervous system, which includes the nerve roots and nerves, is to supply the muscles and various organs within the body.

What connects the brain, spinal cord, and brainstem to the rest of the system are large conduits or nerve bundles, many of which travel relatively long distances between units, such as upper and lower parts of the brain through the spinal cord and back. The basic unit in this communication process, and central to our discussion of psychiatric drugs, is the nerve cell or *neuron*. The action takes place here.

Neurons are connected to each other by means of specific contacts or synapses which appear on two different fibers of the cell, called *axons* and *dendrites*. The system works when chemical messengers or *neurotransmitters* are passed from cell to cell through these synapses. How this exchange takes place is still not very well known. We think that through a series of chemical events that occur at the synapse, the incoming chemical messenger alters the chemical makeup of a secondary messenger. Then that messenger is released to the next cell, which sets off a similar process. Hence, the changes elicited by the messenger at the nerve gaps are reproduced from nerve to nerve, much like a message is passed from person to person in the parlor-game telephone.

How Psychiatric Medications Work

A psychiatric medication affects the central nervous system by either increasing, decreasing, or modulating the concentration of the neurotransmitter chemical at the synapse. For example, what we clinically call depression is thought to be a relative decrease in that part of the central nervous system that uses the chemical messengers *norepinephrine* and *serotonin*. Some antidepressant drugs, therefore, slow down the metabolism or the breakdown of these two messengers, which allows them to remain at the synapse for a longer time. The effect of the drug prolongs the life of the neurotransmitter and, in turn, diminishes or prevents the symptoms of depression.

Another example is the action of an *antipsychotic* medication. Psychosis is thought to be caused by excessive amounts of another neurotransmitter called *dopamine*. It is our understanding that antipsychotic drugs have a positive effect on someone with psychotic symptoms because the drug acts to block or reduce the amount of available dopamine.

Do psychiatric drugs cure or correct? The best way to discuss this complicated issue is with an analogy. If we were to look at the cause of a psychiatric illness as a *mis-wiring* in our nervous system, the role drugs play is to help the body correct the problem. The drug corrects the mis-wiring by affecting the respective neurotransmitter system.

In some instances, however, psychiatric illnesses are recurrent; this implies a permanent *hard-wire* defect. In such a case, the hard-wiring problem is a physiological defect that causes the psychiatric symptoms or behavior. No drug can permanently correct an anatomical defect. Hence, in these more severe cases, the medication may be taken on a long-term or, perhaps, permanent basis in order to continue to correct the problem.

I should point out that this description of the impact of drugs on neurotransmitters is a somewhat limited explanation for the events that we call behavior, particularly symptoms of psychiatric diseases. It is not meant to imply that this explanation or model accounts for all the phenomena that we see. But, broadly speaking, it should be a useful description of how some psychiatric medications probably act on the chemical messengers of the central nervous system to bring about changes in our thinking, feeling, and behavior.

Side Effects

When I am asked by a patient if the drug they are taking will produce many side effects, I feel my answer is not always satisfying. I tell them that many psychiatric drugs produce relatively few side effects; and some, many more.

Primarily, those drugs that act only on a single system within the central nervous system—so-called *clean* drugs—usually produce the fewest side effects, though they are not always less serious or troublesome. On the other hand, those psychiatric drugs that affect multiple systems within the central nervous system usually produce the greatest number of side effects.

The lack of precision in the action of most psychiatric drugs reflects the limited information we have about the brain and how it works. It also reveals the unique complexity of human behavior.

Wanted and Unwanted Effects

The wanted or desired effect of a drug is that which the drug does to address the problem for which it was prescribed. For example, you take an antibiotic to clear up an infection; likewise, an anti-depressant relieves depression. On the other hand, unwanted or undesirable effects are those that occur along with or "on the side" of these intended effects. These unwanted effects are often classified separately as *side effects* and *adverse reactions*. Side effects are thought to be more usual or predictable and less serious. Adverse reactions are less predictable and more serious.

The vast majority of side effects are only a nuisance and usually do not last long. They often occur within the first 72 hours and disappear as your body adjusts to the continued use of the drug. For example, a highly common side effect of many psychiatric medications, dry mouth, usually ceases after a few weeks. If your dosage is increased or decreased, however, you might once again feel a side effect you had when you first started taking the drug, possibly dry mouth or dizziness.

Side effects do not increase in proportion to the length of time you use a drug. The symptoms that appear with extended use are not called side effects, but adverse reactions.

Ironically, the issue of whether a drug's effects are wanted or unwanted may depend upon the circumstances. In one instance, for insomnia, drowsiness may be the wanted effect; in another, it may be only a side effect. It all depends whether the situation or treatment calls for sedation or not. An example of that would be in the multiple uses of antihistamines. BENADRYL (page 222) is an antihistamine prescribed in the treatment of allergies. Among other benefits, it reduces nasal congestion and mucus flow as it dries the lining of the nose; it also causes many people to become drowsy. In these circumstances, the drying sinus is the wanted effect and the drowsiness is the predictable but unwanted side effect.

However, these roles can be reversed. If the antihistamine is taken to treat transitory insomnia, the drowsiness is precisely what you want and the dryness of the nose and throat is its unwanted side effect.

When you are prescribed any medication, you should ask your doctor what the probable side effects are. For example, will you be sleepy for periods during the day? Will the medication affect your appetite? Knowing the most likely or usual side effects in advance will help you develop the necessary confidence in your medication and in your doctor. You may also want to learn a few of the unusual effects or adverse reactions the drug may produce. But if the drug is used properly, most adverse reactions are unlikely to occur; the vast number of them are statistically insignificant: less than 1 percent.

If you find the side effects troubling or they persist for more than a week, see your doctor. He or she can reduce the dosage schedule or substitute another drug from the same drug family. It is because manufacturers are constantly looking to develop more effective drugs that produce fewer and milder side effects that we have many different drugs available for the same condition.

As we will see later, different people develop different side effects for reasons that are as much peculiar to them as to the pharmacological property of the drug. (See Chapter 4, "People at Particular Risk.")

Weight Gain

Tricyclic antidepressants, usually prescribed for depression, frequently produce one of the most exasperating of all the common side effects: increased appetite and subsequent weight gain. In some individuals, the weight gain increases the depression, especially if the underlying disorder is centered on self-rejection. In these instances, drugs such as PROZAC (page 119) and DESYREL (page 118) are preferable in treating atypical depression because they usually diminish appetite and carbohydrate craving.

If you put on unwanted weight while taking lithium, TEGRETOL (page 280) may be an effective substitute; it is rare that someone puts on weight with this drug.

PSYCHIATRIC DRUGS THAT MAY CAUSE WEIGHT GAIN

(In order of greatest potential)

Generic Names

amitriptyline	doxepin	amoxapine
chlorpromazine	imipramine	carbamazepine
lithium	maprotiline	desipramine
mesoridazine	nortriptyline	haloperidol
thioridazine	perphenazine	tranylcypromine
	phenelzine	trazodone
	thiothixene	
	trifluoperazine	

What to Do About Side Effects

The solutions for many minor side effects are simple and practical. Dry mouth, one of the most common side effects, can be irritating. For the elderly, it is especially troubling since it can make swallowing difficult and discourage some elderly people from eating properly. To relieve the symptoms of dry mouth, I suggest you chew sugarless gum, eat a piece of hard candy, or chew on ice chips. They should adequately moisten your mouth.

If your problem is orthostatic hypotension (low blood pressure), with your doctor's supervision, I would suggest you increase your intake of fluids or salt. The value of increasing your salt intake is that it draws in more fluid to your blood system (or increases intervascular volume), which increases the volume of your blood and blood pressure. It is not unlike a garden hose: if you turn on more water, it grows stiffer and increases the pressure in the hose. Increasing the amount of fluids you drink each day will also help add to the blood volume.

If certain medications reduce your ability to fall asleep or stay asleep, take the medication in the morning. Many of my patients find that when they take PROZAC (page 119) or NORPRAMIN (page 103) early in the morning, it doesn't affect their sleep at night.

If your medication affects your sexual performance at night, besides calling your doctor, you might consider taking the drug early in the morning, or take it at night and conduct your sexual activities early in the morning. Whatever the strategy, the key is to increase the interval between the effects of the medication and the sexual act. In some cases, a lower dose may lessen this particular side effect, too.

However, if the effects from the psychiatric drugs you use become troubling—whether they affect breathing, muscular coordination, dizziness, or sexual performance, or if they persist for more than a week—notify your doctor. The persistence and gravity of the symptoms is something your doctor needs to know. Unfortunately, some of my patients, and those of other doctors too, are reluctant to bother me, especially on a weekend. Sometimes they are afraid that their doctor would be angry or impatient over the reasons for the phone call. In return, I say to my patients: "You are always talking about your life. In that regard, there are no stupid or minor questions. In the practice of health care, we share the same goals; but if we do not share the same information, we may undermine those mutual efforts."

Latency Period

Unlike conventional medicines, some psychiatric drugs require a longer period of time before they are effective. This interval is called their *latency* period. An antibiotic, for example, works quickly on controlling the infected site. In the same manner, a diuretic works directly on the kidney to excrete more water. But because psychiatric drugs affect nervous systems within our body, sometimes more than one at a time, it appears that they require a period of readjustment before they can be effective. The latency period is not the same for all psychiatric drugs: some drugs take effect in four to seven days and others require between ten days to two weeks.

When I have failed to make my patients fully understand the phenomenon of a latency period, I will get calls from some of them telling me that they are already experiencing a change for the better, virtually from the first day of their drug use. If they are "benefiting" from the drug, I tell them that this is good news. I also add, however, that the therapeutic result has almost everything to do with their commitment to their therapy and desire for change and nothing to do with the pharmacological qualities of the drug.

In medicine, this phenomenon of beneficial results not caused by the pharmacological properties of a drug is called the *placebo effect*. The placebo effect (*placebo* in Latin means "I shall please") is never a trivial matter. In psychiatric treatment it is therapeutically helpful since it strongly suggests the positive power found in the patient's cooperative attitude. (I mentioned earlier how a patient's unwillingness to get well can, in a parallel manner, *undermine* the effectiveness of psychiatric medication and actually frustrate recovery.) Thus, I always tell my patients that in psychiatric therapy the committed search for help is, in itself, therapeutic.

I will also get calls from some disappointed patients who have lost confidence in their medication because it has not done anything—after only a few days of use. They are upset that they still feel the same and that there has been no change for the better. On some occasions, I will hear from patients that they are experiencing dramatic adverse reactions after only one dose.

In all of these situations, I remind them that the drug generally needs a week or more before it can produce *any* effects. For those people who are frustrated because the drug has not eliminated their symptoms, I assure them that with patience their desire for improvement will be a positive force in their future therapy.

It appears that many of us, however, have very fixed expectations about the efficacy of medications in general. Despite what our doctors might tell us about psychiatric drugs, we hold firmly to the belief that any drug "worth its salt" should begin to produce results within a few days. Hence, after I have presented what I think has been a thorough explanation of psychiatric drug use to my patients, I usually ask them to summarize what I have just told them. I frequently learn that they have not fully understood me and so I repeat the material. I try to be very sympathetic in these situations since many of these people are under stress, which is not the best condition for learning. Also, if we are serious about health-care information, it bears repeating.

Adverse Reactions

It is possible, although less likely, that you will experience drug effects that are more serious than the side effects listed in each of the drug entries of this book. These drug effects, also listed in each drug entry and referred to as *adverse reactions*, are unusual and sometimes harmful. These adverse reactions also include allergic responses to the drug.

Neither side effects nor adverse reactions are signs that you have necessarily received an incorrect medication or dosage for your condition. Both side effects and adverse reactions are part of the legitimate risk each drug poses, albeit a small one. In those instances in which an adverse reaction occurs, if you are being properly supervised by your doctor, the reaction can be handled without serious risk to your health. *When you experience a reaction that is persistent, causing you discomfort—or is a health problem or is not what you believed or were told could happen— then call your doctor.* I say, *call* your doctor because it may be necessary for you to get advice immediately. However, you should not stop taking the drug without your doctor's knowledge; that may cause additional problems (see "Terminating Psychiatric Medication," page 84). You and your doctor should establish a procedure in advance as to how you should handle any of the likely drug reactions associated with the medication you have been prescribed.

Sometimes the most troubling unwanted effects of drug use are those that are totally unexpected, often referred to as *idiosyncratic reactions*. An example is an allergic response to a medication, such as body rash. Not only is an allergic response surprising and dramatic, but it can be very serious. If you develop a skin rash, call your doctor immediately.

It is important to mention here that not all skin rashes are allergic responses. Some drugs are *photo-sensitizing*, that is, they make the skin so sensitive to the sun that a reddish rashlike reaction may develop. This is not the same as an allergic reaction to the drug. If this occurs, stay out of the sun. If you are unsure about the *cause* of the rash, phone your doctor.

Allergies

To reduce the likelihood of allergic responses, it is critical that you tell your doctor of any unusual responses you have had with drugs in the past, both prescription and over-the-counter (OTC). Though you may not recognize the symptoms of a drug-related allergic response, if you have any symptom that is unusual, unexpected, or troublesome, notify your doctor. It need not be the first time you take the drug before an allergic response occurs. Often it is the second exposure to a drug that produces the most distinct and serious allergic response.

People who have a history of allergies—such as hay fever, hives, food allergies, asthma, eczema, and nasal polyps—are more likely to develop an allergic response to drugs. An example of a serious allergic reaction is hepatitis, evidenced by dark urine and a yellowing of the eyes and skin. It's also rare. However, people taking antipsychotic drugs, especially THORAZINE, are exposed to this risk more than with most other drugs.

Another highly disturbing reaction is called a *paradoxical reaction*, a response that is the very opposite of what was intended. Such totally contrary reactions are rare. It seems that they occur more among the elderly, and occasionally in children. For example, a normally sedating drug, such as phenobarbital, might cause an elderly patient to become highly agitated. It's believed that the aging nervous system in some elderly patients produces this response.

Another instance of a paradoxical reaction—but one that is anticipated and intended—occurs with the use of amphetamines in the treatment of children with attention-deficit disorder. These children are usually hyperactive and unable to concentrate or pay attention in school. Unlike other active children, they never seem to stop moving, nothing holds their attention, and they go from one activity to another without completing anything. What is interesting is that the drug to treat the child is a psychostimulant that acts on the developing central nervous system of the child and *paradoxically* causes tranquilization rather than the expected stimulation. It is not clear why these contradictory or paradoxical reactions occur, but it may have something to do with the fact that the nervous systems of these children are still not fully developed.

Extrapyramidal Effects

The side effects or adverse reactions of a psychiatric drug are usually related to the nervous system that the drug acts upon. Major tranquilizers, such as HALDOL (page 160), bring relief primarily by affecting dopamine transmission, and the principal areas affected are the limbic and extrapyramidal systems. These systems are located in the area of the brain that controls the coordination of voluntary movements. Therefore, many of the side effects associated with major tranquilizers are extrapyramidal, that is, they can cause abnormal movements.

These abnormal movements are obvious and bizarre. Some people develop abnormal mouth movements in which they chew vigorously or make searching movements with their tongue; they also make sucking, licking, or lip-pursing movements. Other people experience muscle rigidity, especially stiff back muscles, slowness of movements, and a lack of facial expression. Some other symptoms are a "pill-rolling" motion with their fingers or a hand tremor which is slow and rhythmic in nature. All of these symptoms resemble those of Parkinson's disease and are often referred to as *pseudo-Parkinson's*.

Extrapyramidal symptoms are dose-related, that is, the likelihood of their occurrence is directly related to the amount of the drug taken. Consequently, if you were to experience such symptoms, your doctor would probably either lower your dosage or eliminate the drug altogether. However, your doctor could also find it more appropriate to treat these often disquieting and, occasionally, quite serious extrapyramidal symptoms with other drugs.

Orientals seem to be particularly sensitive to the extrapyramidal side effects of certain psychiatric drugs. We do not know why this is so, but as a result, they tend to require lower doses of those drugs that produce extrapyramidal symptoms than most occidental people.

The medications that are used to treat extrapyramidal symptoms were not originally designed for that purpose but for the treatment of a wide variety of other ailments. SYMMETREL (page 232), for example, belongs to a family of drugs called antivirals— used primarily to prevent or treat flu infections. It also belongs to a family of medications called antidyskinetics since it possesses qualities that are useful in treating extrapyramidal effects or abnormal motor movements, whether brought on by a disease, such as Parkinson's, or the side effects of a psychiatric drug. SYMMETREL also seems effective in treating tardive dyskinesia (see page 292). Its drawback is that, if used in excess, it can induce a state of confusion and, possibly, hallucinations.

BENADRYL is a commonly used antihistamine medication, but it also acts rapidly to correct extrapyramidal effects, especially something called *acute dystonia*, a condition in which someone twists his or her body—neck and head or arms and legs—into abnormal positions. In these cases, BENADRYL is often given intramuscularly to treat the symptoms.

ARTANE (page 230) is another drug that is effective in reducing extrapyramidal symptoms. In this case, the problem is called *akathisia*: a state of constant restlessness. People cannot sit still, and they complain of racing thoughts. Since the drug comes in a form in which it is slowly released in the body, ARTANE is used long term or in maintenance with major tranquilizers. INDERAL (page

266), commonly used for the treatment of high blood pressure, irregular heartbeats, and migraine headaches, is another drug effective in akathisia, as well as treating lithium-induced tremors and tardive dyskinesia.

Again, these are somewhat dramatic drug effects and might be frightening. If they occur, do not hesitate to call your doctor.

Steady-State Blood Level

The goal of a well-managed drug regimen is to establish a consistent and appropriate amount of the drug in your blood system, called a *steady-state blood level*. A uniform amount of the drug in your blood system usually ensures that it will be safe and effective. On the other hand, a dramatic change in your blood level can cause dramatic and unwanted toxic changes.

Some medications, such as LITHIUM, TEGRETOL, NORPRAMIN, and AVENTYL, require regular blood sampling to determine if blood levels are within safe limits. This procedure, usually conducted in a local commercial laboratory or hospital, takes about five minutes and, depending upon the speed of the lab work, the results can be available in a few hours or few days.

One reason LITHIUM needs to be monitored with blood samplings is that at toxic levels it can have an adverse effect on the kidneys. If you are prescribed this drug on a regular or maintenance basis, you should have periodic blood tests and thyroid or heart function tests to make sure that the drug is not adversely affecting these organs. Again, the blood sample is a routine, simple, and safe procedure. It is designed to reassure you and your doctor that your body is handling the drug as it was intended.

Following a Drug Schedule

To achieve a steady-state blood level, most medications have to be given in several doses daily, or *divided doses*, at least initially. We need to gradually build your daily dosage of the drug to the level that delivers the maximum benefits at the lowest risk to you.

When appropriate, the easiest regimen for the divided doses follows the natural divisions of your day: early morning, before or with meals, and before sleep. If the doses are not comfortably placed within your daily routine, your medication program may become a nuisance. A common complaint of many people is that their drug regimen makes them self-conscious, especially if, to protect their privacy, they must surreptitiously excuse themselves at various times of the day to go into the bathroom to take their medication.

Failure to maintain a faithful schedule of medication produces a number of potential problems: principally, the return of symptoms. If this happens, it can cause people to grow discouraged with their entire program of treatment.

It is not always easy to keep to a precise schedule. When people miss a dose, they *make up* for it by doubling the next dose. This is dangerous. The correct policy is this: should you miss a single dose in a multiple-dose regimen, take the next dose at its appointed time. Do not try to compensate or make up for the missed dose by taking more than is indicated. Doubling the dosage only risks creating excessively high blood levels that may produce toxic symptoms. If you immediately return to your normal schedule, without doubling the next dose, the correct blood level will return in an orderly fashion and without any untoward symptoms or harm to you.

If you find being faithful to a particular drug schedule is difficult, ask your doctor to make a change. As you will see, different medications permit different scheduling options for your doctor. For example, depending upon the circumstances, LITHIUM (page 276) may be needed as often as four times a day or only twice a day. Better yet, the antidepressant PROZAC is a drug that need be taken only once a day—in the morning or before going to bed. Because PROZAC has a long half-life, that is, it lasts longer in the body than other drugs, it's possible that someone need only take it every other day. Finally, depot drugs (see page 177) can be administered in a single, deep, intramuscular injection as infrequently as once a week to twice a month.

Your drug schedule is something you and your doctor should work together on. Among other things, ascertain which drug regimen works best for your particular life-style and habits. In some cases, your doctor may have to wait until the symptoms have been brought under control before he or she can offer a drug regimen that works best with the least amount of inconvenience. But drug scheduling options almost always exist.

Causes of Psychiatric Symptoms

Many people fail to understand that the origin of many symptoms is not always obvious—even to a psychiatrist. For example, the cause of a psychiatric symptom may be either physiological or psychological, or both. Being able to differentiate between these two possible causes, obviously, is an absolute requirement before correctly treating the problem.

An uncommon but not rare ailment is an underactive thyroid gland, called *hypothyroidism*. Hypothyroidism, characterized by a slowing down of all your body processes, produces symptoms such as lethargy, constipation, weight gain, and feelings of depression. These are also many of the same symptoms associated with a psychological disorder, such as grief or extended mourning.

The following are two examples of how certain symptoms might be understandably misinterpreted by someone who is not trained to make the necessary distinction.

Some years ago, a man came to me and said that he thought his seventy-year-old mother needed psychiatric help. During the past six months, she was gradually becoming more anxious at night. He became deeply concerned when her complaints included seeing apparitions at night. His mother also said she heard mutterings or conversations that were menacing or threatening.

When he brought her in to see me the next week, I met an intelligent woman who was obviously very worried that she was going crazy. After a physical examination, however, I learned that she was anything but crazy. She was suffering from cataracts which were progressively clouding her vision, making her world grayer and mistier—and somewhat more threatening-looking, I suppose. In addition, this woman was developing a hardening of the muscles of the middle ear, which accounted for her faulty hearing. Consequently, when evening approached or when the general level of light was diminished in a room, her impaired senses caused her to imagine she was seeing and hearing something else. Her growing sense of apprehension was probably also fed by the fact that she lived alone.

Within two weeks, a simple surgical procedure that corrected the cataracts and a hearing aid solved this woman's "psychiatric" symptoms.

The other case involved a much younger woman. A thirty-four-year-old single woman with a brief history of psychotherapy (while a student in college) came to me with all the symptoms of general anxiety. She had a periodic tremor, was nervous and anxious, and was noticeably perspiring. She also fell into a stare at various times of the day. Jokingly, she said that the only good news was that she was losing weight.

Again, although these physical symptoms appeared to be classical psychiatric signs of anxiety, a physical examination revealed a different diagnosis. She had what is technically referred to as Grave's disease. Her symptoms were the direct result of an overactive thyroid—*hyperthyroidism.*

As you can see, the possible causes of psychiatric symptoms may point in several different directions, and the symptoms may not even be psychiatric in nature. In my view, the most appropriate health-care professional to interpret such symptoms, make a correct diagnosis, and recommend an appropriate and effective course of treatment is a psychiatrist, who is, of course, a trained medical doctor as well.

In addition to physiological causes, we have learned over the past three or four decades that psychological trauma, such as early loss of parents, death of a spouse, or socioeconomic hardship, can cause psychological and physiological symptoms that can be both severe and long-lasting. Certain catastrophic events, for example, cause the kinds of profound symptoms that lead to serious dys-functioning. For example, I have seen many Vietnam veterans who suffered from what is sometimes called the *post-traumatic stress syndrome*, that is, a cluster of symptoms that include an overreac-tion to loud noises, general nervousness, and wariness. Many of these people also had a variety of physical ailments. My point is that psychological events can produce, jointly, powerful psycho-logical and physiological symptoms.

The psychological cause need not be catastrophic. The tension caused by chronic interpersonal stress, such as a failing marriage or a dying parent, can generate various psychiatric symptoms ranging from anxiety to depression. I find that people who are intensely emotional—for example, those whose relationships with their parents have been marked over the years by passions that ranged from feelings of hatred to idealized adoration—are people who experience frequent and recurring psychiatric symptoms.

When talking about possible causes of psychiatric symptoms or disorders, a patient will occasionally ask the importance of inborn or genetically transmitted defects versus external and environmen-tal triggers. In other words, which is the more common cause of psychiatric disorders: what you are "born with" or what you "pick up"? My answer is always the same: depending upon the circumstances, either one or both.

Some psychiatric disorders appear to have a genetic or inher-ited component, yet it is not always easy to determine if someone is at a *genetic risk* since there is reason to believe that both a genetic predisposition and an environmental opportunity or exposure are necessary for any particular disorder to occur. People may be born with a propensity for a particular disorder, but this does not mean that the disorder will actually develop.

For example, the risk for major depressions, phobic disorders, or chemical-abuse disorders (such as alcoholism) may be carried from one generation to another. But it does not follow that every-one in any one family will have the genetic disposition or, if so, will exhibit its symptoms. Just because parents may be alcoholics or drug abusers, it does not mean that any or all of their children will be. In addition to the genetic susceptibility, there seems to be some form of complex variable, an action which we do not as yet fully understand, that is necessary for the appearance of the psychiatric illness. For example, even though someone may have a genetic risk factor for a certain psychiatric disorder, there needs to be some other event (such as a medical illness) to trigger the symptoms of psychiatric disorder. If there is no trigger, that person will not experience the disorder.

What role can psychiatric drugs play in these hereditary situations? In these circumstances, psychiatric drugs work as a corrective—not a curative. Some inherited disorders are intermittent, that is, they occur periodically. An effective psychiatric drug will compensate for the genetic flaw by acting as a corrective and reduce or prevent the recurrence of the symptoms.

ALCOHOLISM AND GENES

An example of the complex relationship between psychiatric illnesses and genes can be observed in the discovery of a particular gene strongly associated with alcoholism.

Recent studies have established a link between a particular gene defect and a chronic deficit of the neurotransmitter, dopamine. The potential significance of this connection is that dopamine levels are related to several psychiatric disorders, some of which may be associated with the compulsion to abuse alcohol.

This finding is obviously extremely speculative, but it does add another possible link in the complex association of a genetic defect that is carried from one generation to another and a specific biochemical phenomenon. Again, we are far from recognizing the bridge between genetic risks and the onset of psychological illness; but such discoveries do make us more aware of the possibilities of a shared risk within a single family.

For example, if one member of a family suffers from a major depression or symptoms of a recurrent panic disorder, other family members—both siblings and members of the next generation—could be, in a sense, at risk. In these cases, we might be able to prevent or diminish the problem through the use of different therapies. If a recurrent psychiatric disease is already active in a family, recognizing its genetic cause can be helpful in making a diagnosis and in the choice of treatment. Sometimes, just knowing about its genetic roots makes it easier for people to cope with the troubling mystery or guilt they may feel about the presence of a particular psychiatric disorder in their family. However, despite this greater awareness of a genetic link to certain psychiatric disorders, there is finally very little research to support a case for a predictable cause-and-effect connection.

Another cause of psychiatric symptoms or illnesses may be certain events or anatomical changes that occurred during fetal development or at birth. The consequences of these "silent" events may only show up later in some form of aberrant behavior, such as odd or bizarre thinking (as in the case of schizophrenia). A more obvious link is found in the necessity for prenatal care. In the past twenty years we have learned the impact of the mother's health and life-style on the health of the fetus—especially with regard to drug use. For example, a pregnant woman who drinks heavily risks giving birth to a child with fetal alcohol syndrome (FAS), a condition that produces birth defects that affect its physical and mental growth and include a wide variety of psychiatric symptoms and disorders. (See "Pregnant and Lactating Women," page 66.)

Once again, I have made a somewhat arbitrary division of psychiatric diseases of the central nervous system that are *organic*—illnesses which are caused by some structural or physiological change in the brain—and illnesses that are strictly *psychological*—disorders which are not seemingly a product of any physiological or biochemical change. I say the distinction is arbitrary or, at least, not very precise because all psychological events produce a physiological response—when you are depressed you have physical signs of depression. Nevertheless, the distinction of whether a disorder is organic or psychological in origin is important because the choice of treatment your doctor recommends will be governed by what he or she believes has caused the disorder.

THREE

Common Psychiatric Disorders

Psychiatric drugs are used to treat many forms of mental illness or affective disorders because the chemistry of the brain plays an important part in causing them. However, any comprehensive list or thorough discussion of the various mental illnesses for which psychiatric drugs are prescribed would be too lengthy and complex for this handbook. If you are interested in learning more about such serious psychiatric illnesses as manic depression, schizophrenia, and Korsakoff's syndrome, I suggest you consult a more specialized book that deals in-depth with the treatment of these disorders. Of course, before undertaking any reading on a particular illness, you should first ask the physician who is treating you those basic questions you need answered. After speaking to your doctor, you might be better able to identify what kind of book or materials would be most helpful to you.

The disorders I have chosen to discuss here are those that affect the largest number of people on a daily basis. They are the most common mental health problems I see in my practice and for which my patients have the greatest curiosity. Because they are commonly discussed, I find that there is a good deal of confusion or misinformation associated with them. Nevertheless, most of these disorders can today be treated successfully and with little or no discomfort.

Insomnia

More than half of my patients come to me with complaints of irregular sleep habits. They believe that, initially, their unconventional or abnormal sleep patterns are connected with their other psychiatric symptoms, such as anxiety or depression—and they often are.

Although their sleep habits may be a sign of insomnia, I point out to my patients that there is no standard sleep pattern by which someone can judge if they are sleeping normally. Very healthy people have sleep habits that consist of only five hours of sleep every night while others will require nine- or ten-hour sleep periods. So, the amount of sleep will vary widely from one person to another. What is important, however, is if people are rested or refreshed after their sleep.

Hence, even though sleep needs vary widely, it is still relatively easy to identify or define insomnia. I use the term *insomnia* to mean insufficient or nonrestorative sleep. Common sleep behaviors—such as difficulty falling asleep, staying asleep, sleeping deeply enough, or sleeping long enough into the morning—can be signs of insomnia. Without regard to your sleep patterns, however, if you are consistently unable to get enough rest at night to keep you alert during a normal day, then it can be said that you are probably suffering from insomnia.

Insomnia is usually situational and time-limited: that is, it is triggered by specific situations and usually doesn't last more than a few weeks or months. It is a symptom that affects 20 to 40 percent of all people using psychiatric drugs. It afflicts women more than men, usually people in the higher socioeconomic classes, and it increases with age. For about 17 percent of everyone affected by insomnia, it develops into a chronic problem.

Insomnia is usually due to (1) an illness, (2) a medication, or (3) a psychological cause. If caused by an illness—that is, if the symptoms of your illness awaken you, such as difficult breathing, recurrent pain, or attacks of severe indigestion—then the treatment of the illness and its symptoms will, in effect, treat the insomnia. If your medications, whether psychiatric or conventional, alter your sleep, you should notify your doctor. A wide variety of medications, both prescription and nonprescription, can disturb sleep because they contain stimulants. If the sleep disorder is due to anxiety or tension associated with an event or something else in your life, a limited use of specific medications and sleep practices commonly solves the problem.

Insomnia is not uniform; sometimes it is not serious; at other times it can be very troubling. It is also highly subjective since the experience of sleep differs from person to person. However, the relative seriousness of the disorder can be divided generally into three categories:

1. *Transient* insomnia is usually caused by external events, such as a change of environment (e.g., so-called jet lag) or an anticipation of a coming event. It usually lasts only a few days.
2. *Short-term* insomnia is caused by pharmacological agents, such as stimulants (e.g., coffee, nicotine, and alcohol), by the side effect of certain medications, as well as by traumatizing events, such as the loss of a job. Short-term insomnia lasts longer than transitory insomnia—usually a few weeks.
3. *Long-term* or *chronic* insomnia is usually defined as insomnia that lasts longer than three weeks. A diagnosis of chronic insomnia should take into consideration not only the onset of the insomnia but its duration and history. For example, I always want to know if the insomnia is constant or if it comes and goes, if vivid dreaming is involved, and when the last time someone had at least one week of restorative sleep. Equally important is whether he or she is taking any medications, including alcohol, or has had a history of drug abuse.

Long-term insomnia most often is related to a physical illness, especially one associated with an infection or pain, or a psychiatric illness, such as depression. Examples of other psychiatric disorders that commonly cause long-term insomnia are anxiety (associated with a generalized anxiety disorder), panic disorders, and obsessive-compulsive thinking. Again, in these cases your insomnia would be viewed and treated as a symptom of a larger illness. The drug selected for the specific illness may eliminate the symptom causing the insomnia, such as pain, or the drug may have some sedating properties that will help induce sleep.

If your insomnia is diagnosed as a primary sleep disorder, such as *sleep apnea*, it will require careful evaluation and treatment by a specialist.

Most sleep medications usually lose their effectiveness after three to four weeks. When you stop using such a drug, especially after taking it for more than four weeks, do it gradually over a period of about a week. If you abruptly stop your use of the sleep medication, you may have insomnia for a period, including vivid and disturbing dreams. This phenomenon called *rebound insomnia* occurs because, during the time you have used the medication, your body has grown accustomed or become adapted to its presence. If the drug is suddenly withdrawn, your body may not be able to immediately adjust to its absence. What happens, then, is a relapse into the same or worse symptoms of insomnia—at least temporarily. Therefore, when terminating a sleep medication, especially a prescription drug, notify your doctor, who can also advise you how to properly discontinue its use.

Benzodiazepines (such as DALMANE, RESTORIL, or HALCION) are the most suitable drugs for producing a sleep that most closely approximates the natural state that leaves you refreshed. But these drugs generally have high dependency qualities. Consequently, they should be given in a closely monitored, symptom-targeted, and time-limited fashion. Even though you will probably find that after approximately two weeks they may begin to lose their effectiveness, by no means should you continue to use them for more than a month. If your insomnia persists, notify your doctor for a change in treatment.

Moreover, open-ended or refillable prescriptions should never be given for these drugs, and they should not be terminated abruptly or taken in conjunction with alcohol. Because they have sedating qualities, some antihistamines and NOCTEC (page 202) can be safe and effective for inducing sleep.

On the other hand, SECONAL (page 196) may induce sleep but the sleep will not be physiologically or psychologically restorative: that is to say, you will probably wake up tired or weary or with a hangover. If you are consistently troubled by waking early, it may be a sign of depression, a disorder which can be made worse by the use of hypnotic drugs. If you experience a continuous pattern of unexplained insomnia, see your doctor. A prudent medical and psychological evaluation can determine its cause.

I often see people who have developed something called *anticipatory insomnia*: the more they try to sleep, the less they are able to. As they anticipate being sleepless, convinced they probably will not fall asleep, they aggravate their insomnia. In these situations (and they all differ), I frequently recommend taking a nonprescription sleep aid for a few days, such as an antihistamine which makes you drowsy. I also recommend that they consider the following sleep hygiene practices since I continue to be surprised at how little attention people give to good sleep practices. Of course, not all cases of insomnia, short- or long-term, respond to these steps, but they are often helpful:

1. Get up and go to bed at approximately the same times each day—including weekends. Your body anticipates sleep at relatively scheduled periods and any change in that rhythm may result in a less refreshing sleep.
2. Use the bed and pillow only to sleep. It should not be used for reading, watching television, or working.
3. Avoid napping during the day.
4. Exercise regularly, but not in the evening.

5. Reduce your consumption of alcohol, nicotine, and caffeine.
6. If you cannot fall asleep, do not remain in bed longer than twenty to thirty minutes. Leave the bedroom and do not return until you are drowsy.

Note: There may be a biochemical basis to the time-honored practice of parents giving their children cookies and milk at bedtime to help them get to sleep. Milk, along with many foods containing animal and fish protein, contains the amino acid *tryptophan*. Tryptophan, which serves as a precursor for serotonin, a chemical important in nerve transmission and sedation, can be useful in very small amounts in inducing safe, natural sleep.

Some years ago tryptophan was recommended to people in tablet form to treat insomnia. However, it is generally no longer available in health food stores or pharmacies since, in many cases, its prolonged use had lead to an occurrence of *eosinophilia myalgia syndrome*, an inflammation of small blood vessels in the muscles that results in soreness and atrophy or loss of muscle tissue.

In summary, *sleeping pills* are only a temporary solution and should be used only occasionally and for short periods. If insomnia persists despite your best efforts to cure it, see your doctor.

NONPRESCRIPTION SLEEP AIDS

Read the labels of your over-the-counter sleep aids.

The FDA has determined that products containing diphenhydramine and doxylamine are safe and effective nonprescription sleep aids. These compounds are antihistamines and act on the central nervous system to cause drowsiness. Consequently, they are used to induce sleepiness or to maintain sleep through the night. However, the FDA considers all other nonprescription products, including those containing pyrilamine, ineffective as sleep aids.

Some nonprescription sleep aids also contain pain relievers, such as acetaminophen or aspirin, which makes them effective in treating insomnia due to minor pain. It should be noted, however, that although acetaminophen is a pain reliever like aspirin, it does not have the anti-inflammatory or antirheumatic qualities of aspirin.

Depression

Depression, in all its forms, is a common disorder. Basically, it is a *syndrome* (a group of symptoms or disorders) that may have many different or possible causes. Its symptoms can range from sadness, disappointment, and a passing sense of loss to social withdrawal, abject hopelessness, and suicide.

Depression results when one or more of the different systems within the central nervous system—usually the norepinephrine and serotonin systems—fails to function properly. An antidepressant drug acts by increasing the supply of these chemical neurotransmitters. Once restored to normal levels, the depression usually disappears.

The depression most people experience is transient, and usually disappears in a few days or weeks. Studies suggest that about 6 percent of the American population would describe themselves as having depressions. What the general public might consider depression, however, ranges from this transitory depression to more serious or long-lasting symptoms of depression.

Serious depression not only lasts longer but it can make someone quite incapacitated, and it always requires treatment. Proba-

SLEEP TRAVEL

By and large: when traveling eastward (into the sun), your recovery time is one day for every time zone. It takes slightly *less* than one day when traveling westward, or with the sun.

bly less than 10 percent of those people who report experiencing depression suffer from a clinical or diagnosable depression that requires treatment. Unfortunately, only about one-third of these people who are clinically depressed actually seek or receive treatment. In effect, hundreds of thousands of people probably suffer some form of serious, but untreated, depression.

Serious depression comes in many different forms: for our purposes, we will discuss *secondary, endogenous* (biological in origin), and *reactive* depressions.

Secondary Depression

Secondary depression is caused by a physical disease. One example is hypothyroidism or an underfunctioning thyroid gland. Since virtually all our metabolic processes are affected by the hormones produced by the thyroid gland, if too little are produced, everything in the body slows down. Symptoms of hypothyroidism are lethargy, weight gain or loss of appetite, and the feeling of depression. Once the disorder is corrected, however, the symptoms are relieved, including the depression. Secondary depression may also accompany prolonged use of alcohol or any other central nervous system depressant. (Alcoholism can also be related to anxiety and panic attacks.)

Another disease associated with secondary depression is neoplasm or cancer. The psychiatric symptoms of these cancers, especially cancers located in the pancreas and lungs, include depressive symptoms. Of course, fears associated with its life-threatening possibilities also induce depression.

Endogenous Depression

These recurrent depressions often occur in cycles either by themselves or are linked with manic episodes in a recognizable pattern. Endogenous depressions can also be linked to panic disorders, phobias, and alcoholism, and their frequency usually grows with age. These depressions often have a genetic component.

As I mentioned before, a genetically based depression is a kind of *hard-wiring* problem. An anatomical or genetic defect causes the depression and, since we cannot permanently correct this *hard-wire defect*, some people must take medication for long periods, sometimes lifelong, in order to maintain a proper functioning system.

The permanent use of a drug should not be seen as distressing or drastic. People with essential hypertension (high blood pressure, for example) take a medication on a permanent basis, usually at minimum doses. The drug does not permanently correct or cure the cause of the problem but it prevents the recurrence of the high blood pressure. Among psychiatric disorders, perhaps up to 10 percent of all people taking drugs for severe psychiatric disorders are on some kind of a permanent drug regimen—many of them functioning quite normally.

Hence, people with genetic depression often take a medication for years, or permanently. Medications for this type of depression do not guarantee that there will be no more depressive symptoms. Life events—such as dying, sickness, and other forms of stress—can provoke symptoms. But, if the maintenance drug is unable to prevent any recurrence, it can certainly reduce the frequency and intensity of any possible symptoms. In this respect, the psychiatric medication currently available is generally successful with genetically based depressions.

Over the years I have treated a number of people who suffered from a type of depression—possibly biologically based—called *seasonal affective disorder* (SAD), that is, a disorder that causes people to grow progressively more depressed with the loss of seasonal daylight. In other words, in the fall their depression would begin, grow worse in the winter, and diminish in early spring. By the end of April, they would have no symptoms.

Most of these patients respond to the use of antidepressants. Another treatment for this seasonal disorder usually includes a recently developed procedure called *phototherapy*. In this therapy, people with SAD or other light-dependent depressive disorders are exposed two or three hours in an artificially well-lighted room during the day. Sometimes it is necessary to repeat the therapy once a week during the winter months. Phototherapy is well-received because it is not only effective in those cases in which the depressive symptoms are not severe, but it avoids the unnecessary use of psychiatric drugs.

Reactive Depression

A far more common form of depression is *reactive* depression, which can be transient or develop into a clinical depression. As its name implies, this depression is a reaction to an event or change in a person's life, usually a loss. For example, periods of change or transition, such as the end of schooling or a pregnancy (*postpartum depression*), or certain chronological milestones, such as turning fifty or retiring, are associated with reactive depression.

Symptoms of Depression

There is no *one* syndrome or pattern of symptoms that is exclusively depression. People exhibit their own particular and peculiar patterns of symptoms. Depression includes symptoms of sadness, loss of energy and motivation, backward-looking or second-guessing one's self, and self-deprecation. In the most severe form, hopelessness is the critical symptom. Other manifestations are social withdrawal, loss of appetite, weight loss, sleep disturbances (particularly early-morning wakening) or interrupted sleep, distractibility, and difficulty concentrating.

There are a number of depressive symptoms that are called *atypical* because they are the opposite of the more usual depressive symptoms. For example, many people diagnosed with depression have reported to me that they experienced increased appetite, weight, and need for sleep (*hypersomnulance*).

Depressive symptoms can also appear in a *disguised* form, such as musculoskeletal or arthritic pain and recurrent headaches. Other examples of disguised depressive symptoms may be a change in social habits, particularly an increase in the frequency and amount of alcohol consumed, or the sudden onset of drug abuse.

In young children, depression is seen in symptoms of withdrawal and accident-proneness, and in adolescents, in antisocial behavior and other forms of disruptive behavior.

Besides medication, therapies for depression include phototherapy, electroconvulsive or shock therapy for the more severe cases, and sleep deprivation. The latter proves to be effective for some people in the treatment of their depression because it produces antidepressive qualities.

Whatever the choice of possible therapies, I find that usually the best treatment for depression is a combination of medication and psychotherapy. Besides providing support and education for the use of the medication, psychotherapy can provide a context in which people can better learn which factors in their lives increase their vulnerability to depression. For example, many of the depressed people I treat are initially unable to express their angry feelings. They also need to learn how to express these feelings without resorting to uncontrolled, angry outbursts. Angry or hostile feelings that remain unexpressed become trapped. It is common for people with depression to direct these trapped feelings of anger at *themselves*—only to produce or aggravate their symptoms of depression.

Psychotherapy can help people think and act more effectively on solutions to those external problems in their lives that may contribute to their depression. People with depression may gain from others who can patiently listen to their concerns.

Obsessive-Compulsive Disorders

An obsessive-compulsive disorder (OCD) is a psychiatric disorder characterized by the persistent reappearance of images or impulses, or repetitive behaviors that a person feels driven to perform. I do not mean those minor obsessions or repeated behaviors that may be irrational but do not interfere with your normal life. I am referring to people who, for example, are so fearful of being contaminated that they interrupt their work schedules continually to wash their hands, maybe hourly. These people may wash so vigorously that they excoriate or wear off their skin. They may even choose to wear gloves all day. Another group is called *checkers*, people who habitually are unable to assure themselves that the stove, lights, doors are not *on* or *open*. Hence, they feel forced to check them, sometimes at great inconvenience to themselves and their families. The remaining type of obsessive-compulsive consists of those people with pure obsessional thoughts, usually of a sexual and aggressive nature.

Obsessive-compulsive behaviors vary, but they are recognizable. Generally they are all extremely time-consuming, interfere with one's normal routine, and although they are irrational and purposeless, any attempt to resist them usually leads to increased anxiety. The incidence of OCD is also relatively rare, with no more than 2 percent of the population affected.

Until recently, the only treatment for obsessive-compulsive disorders had been psychotherapy. But now, with effective antidepressant drugs available, such as PROZAC (page 119) and ANAFRANIL (page 122), in conjunction with psychotherapy, treatment of the obsessive-compulsive disorders is more successful and less disruptive for the individual. When used with psychotherapy, ANAFRANIL has been effective in about two-thirds of people treated, and sometimes within a period of three to six weeks.

Its principal side effects are anticholinergic, namely symptoms such as dry mouth, blurred vision, urinary retention, and increased sweating. The one major reservation that I have about ANAFRANIL is its incidence of seizures, although it occurs in less than 1 percent of all persons who take this drug. Like PROZAC, which has also been found to be effective in obsessive-compulsive disorders, the action of the drug increases the availability of serotonin by blocking its reuptake, which means it remains at the synapse longer.

Anxiety

The term *anxiety*, as it is used in psychiatry, has multiple meanings. Basically, anxiety is a description of an uneasiness of the mind, often in an anticipation of an event or an unwanted feeling, such as panic or irrational fear. It may be a symptom associated with depression or a panic attack, or a general disorder of its own. Most people accept brief periods of tension (or anxiety) as part of life's experience. However, if it makes it difficult or impossible for us to live a normal life, then it needs to be treated.

In therapy, I find it beneficial to work with the following distinction between fear and anxiety: fear is a reaction to a clear and present danger, and anxiety is a fearful reaction to an unconscious provocation.

Several years ago a patient of mine first came to me complaining that he was "riddled with anxiety" over the probable failure of his marriage. This anxiety was interfering with his appetite, sleep, and his job as a trial lawyer. His concern was that his anxiety was inappropriate or exaggerated. I reassured him that anxiety is appropriate when a marriage fails, especially when it is one that is as important as his was to him. But only after we spoke further did I realize that his marriage was not in jeopardy, certainly not so much as he thought it might be. In fact, his wife had never mentioned anything about divorce; she had asked him to see a psychiatrist about his anxiety. It turned out that his anxiety was related to a deeper problem of depression which he had lived with most of his life. Poor energy levels, occasional loss of appetite, and career changes were its earlier symptoms. The anxiety, thought at first to be related to his marriage, was only the latest but most intense sign of a developing illness that obviously needed to be treated. His marriage, I might add, survived the treatment; his depression did not.

What is important to understand, then, is that anxiety requires treatment if it persists, causes you to deny the existence of a problem that clearly requires a solution or helpful response, poses a threat to your health (i.e., postcardiac patient), or disables by continually disrupting your normal life.

Anxiety shows up at various times of our lives and in different forms:

1. *Acute anxiety* is usually associated with a sudden onset of an event or some internal conflict which is transient in nature.
2. *Anticipatory anxiety* occurs in panic and phobic disorders, in sleep disorders (anticipation of insomnia), and in anticipation of musculoskeletal pain.
3. *Generalized form of anxiety* is a particular illness in which people experience anxiety for long periods of time. In addition to being a primary illness, it may accompany another illness, such as depression or alcoholism.

Symptoms of Anxiety

The symptoms of anxiety can be categorized as either *objective* or *cognitive*. Objective symptoms are physically apparent: excessive sweating, heart palpitations, racing pulse, fainting, flushes, chills, diarrhea, or stomach cramps. Cognitive symptoms (which are unseen and perhaps more important) include extreme feelings of dying or going crazy.

It is not clear what precipitates or triggers an anxiety syndrome. The anxiety may surface as a generalized anxiety disorder, that is, as a sudden and totally unexplained onset of morbid fear or a panic attack. For example, someone might unexpectedly think and feel that they were going to die—for no apparent reason. It is not unusual for someone suffering from anxiety to become fearful or anxious over a common situation or object, one not normally considered fearful, such as an unexpected and paralyzing fear of crowds or a subway train.

Anxiety is also a component of other psychiatric disorders, such as obsessive-compulsive disorders and panic disorders, which we will discuss later.

We do not completely understand the physiology of anxiety, namely, what the specific biological basis of the illness or symptoms is. At the moment, three chemicals or nervous systems have been implicated: norepinephrine, serotonin, and the gamma-aminobutyric acid (GABA) system. (The complex neurotransmission system of the brain involves many different chemicals that transfer signals from and to nerve cells. These are three of the four chemical systems we best understand. For more information on the central nervous system, see page 28.)

Antianxiety medications that play a role in improving anxiety affect each of these three systems by either increasing, decreasing, or modulating the neurotransmitter or chemical involved. The change in the chemical changes your mood.

As with most psychiatric disorders, there is much to learn about anxiety. What we do know, however, is that if you feel the symptom should be treated, see a health-care professional. This is a problem for which you should be medicated.

If you experience periodic or transient anxiety, I suggest you adopt a stress-reduction practice that you find relaxing. There are many reliable methods of relaxation, not the least of which is transcendental meditation and deep-breathing exercises. These various exercises are not demanding and can be very rewarding and practical.

One exercise I recommend is deep breathing. Most of us are shallow breathers; we use only about one-third of our lung capacity. By breathing more deeply, at least for the brief period of a five-minute exercise, you can grow more relaxed. The following exercise is an example:

1. Sit down and get comfortable. Shake your arms and legs for a few seconds as if releasing muscle tension.
2. Breathe deeply, drawing in the cool air slowly. Relax your stomach and then let it expand; then fill your lungs with air. Swallow, as if locking the fresh oxygen in your lungs, and hold it in for a few seconds. Now exhale slowly, allowing all your muscles to relax, especially

your neck, shoulders, and back. Repeat as often as con-
venient.

The best thing about relaxation exercises is that they permit
you to control your anxiety. They are also discrete and almost
always feasible. Anything other than transient anxiety, however,
should be considered serious, possibly requiring professional help.

Phobic Reactions

Phobias are unreasonable fears that are often chronic and can last
for years or a lifetime. Generally a phobic reaction is intensely
obsessive. People may have an unrealistic fear of a common object
or situation, or their fears may be aroused through a possible
separation. For example, a child is afraid of going to school. If this
fear is actually phobic, it would be considered a fear of separation
from the parent. On the other hand, people with agoraphobia
(fear of open spaces) suffer from a form of separation anxiety in
that their acute fear of public places makes them not want to be
separated from the safety of their home.

Phobic reactions, and especially panic attacks, can also be part
of anxiety syndromes. If sufficiently intense, for example, the
anxiety of the phobia can cause panic (see page 64).

However, many commonplace phobias (such as a fear of
heights or a fear of driving) do *not* require psychiatric treatment.
Two of my patients who live in the New York City area have had a
lifelong fear of driving. Neither has felt the need to treat the fear, if
only because they do not need to drive. They take subways, buses,
and taxis. If, however, their circumstances were to change so that
they had to drive a car, treatment might be in order.

Another example is the fear of heights. The best treatment is to
stay away from high places. Avoidance is a fully appropriate
strategy for dealing with mildly phobic situations. Again, it is only
when a phobic reaction prevents someone from living a relatively
free and normal life that treatment is truly necessary.

Another common form of phobic reaction is claustrophobia (fear of closed spaces). It is conceivable that 20 percent of the readers of this book have experienced at some time in their lives a fear of closed spaces, whether in an elevator, a tunnel, or an airplane. Mild claustrophobic responses are very common and do not require treatment. But if someone were so fearful that he or she could not live or work in a building with elevators, ride in an automobile, or fly in an airplane—as a part of their normal living pattern—it would be essential for them to seek psychiatric help.

Agoraphobia can be an especially devastating phobia, and chronic agoraphobia has made people virtual prisoners in their own houses because they could not control their feelings of fear and panic. This disorder always needs to be treated with psychiatric help.

In addition to psychotherapy, certain phobias have responded well to behavior-modification therapies, such as *desensitization*. For example, by returning the patient imaginatively to the fearful situation, therapists are able to teach people to cope more effectively with their anxieties and fears. Some therapies also involve taking people into the actual situation—e.g., in an airplane or an elevator that does not move—in order to build self-confidence.

Panic Reactions

People who have intense attacks of fear and anxiety, such as claustrophobia or agoraphobia, are said to suffer from panic reactions. In effect, a panic reaction is a severe form of the phobic anxiety.

Panic attacks are usually situational and time-limited. They are triggered by an external event and disappear as soon as the provoking circumstances no longer pose a threat.

Panic reactions are also episodic in nature and usually occur in people who are experiencing stress. A history of recurrent panic attacks may run in the family; that is to say, the disorder can be familial.

Anxiety can be very severe during a panic attack, and people can experience heart palpitations, extreme dizziness, and excessive sweating. Several of my patients have gone to hospital emergency rooms believing they were suffering from a heart attack.

The most effective drugs for treating people with panic attacks are tricyclic antidepressants (pages 97–117). I have had success using these depressants along with short-acting benzodiazepines (pages 260–266) if the person is suffering from *anticipatory anxiety*, also known as performance anxiety. The treatment—involving both psychotherapy and psychiatric medication—takes time, perhaps years, especially if the patient has had a long history of panic attacks. But people who suffer from agoraphobia and other forms of phobias or panic attacks should expect that with proper treatment, their symptoms will diminish over time or even completely disappear, and they will then function freely and normally.

FOUR

People at Particular Risk

I always stress with my patients that, although everyone taking psychiatric drugs is statistically at risk of some side effects or adverse reactions, serious symptoms are not likely and most are rare. Moreover, the likelihood of any one side effect's occurrence varies with each drug and each person. However, predictably, some groups of people are at greater risk of side effects and adverse reactions than others and for different reasons. For example, the developing fetus of a pregnant woman, the low body weight and sensitive growth periods of children, and the delicate health and metabolism of the elderly or people in poor health make them all especially sensitive to the effects of many or most psychiatric drugs. Therefore, these people should consult closely with their doctor before and while taking psychiatric medications.

Pregnant and Lactating Women

The placenta of a pregnant woman is very sensitive to drugs present in the mother's body. The placenta permits various nutrients and hormones to cross through its barrier to nourish the developing fetus. The selective barrier of the placenta also screens out many of those substances that might be harmful to the fetus. It cannot, however, shield the fetus from drugs of the smallest molecular weight. Unfortunately, most psychiatric medicines fall into this category of drugs that can cross into the placenta.

At different stages of pregnancy, the fetus's vulnerability changes. The first three months of pregnancy may be the most critical. During this period (in which the fetus goes through its most exacting and complex period of growth and development and its various organs are being formed), many different drugs could threaten their delicate development. A pregnant woman should avoid, whenever possible, taking most psychiatric drugs during her first trimester.

The principal growth period of the child occurs during the fourth to sixth month of pregnancy, the second trimester. An injudicious use of many psychiatric medications during this trimester could potentially impair its growth, though the child is qualifiably less frail than during its first three months.

During the seventh to ninth months, in which preparation is made for labor and delivery, some potent psychiatric drugs could affect the quality of the mother's labor or the health of the child. The risk of drugs to the health of the fetus, therefore, is at its highest during the first trimester, and drops gradually during the second and third trimesters.

It is important for you to be careful not to become pregnant while taking psychiatric drugs, or for a period of time immediately after you stop taking them. Many psychiatric drugs require a period of abstinence or *washout* period before your body is completely free of any traces of the drug. If you happen to become pregnant during this required washout period, the fetus could still be at risk. The safest procedure, then, is to stop taking any psychiatric medication one to two months before conceiving or at least before your intention to conceive. If there is any doubt that you have become pregnant while taking a psychiatric medication, consult with your doctor about discontinuing the drug. Do not begin taking the medication again until it has been established whether you have conceived.

If you have become pregnant while taking psychiatric drugs, it does not mean that the health of your child is at serious risk. Statistically, the risk of any complication is relatively small, even rare. However, do not resume the medication during the first trimester and, even then, use only drugs that are known to be safe under those circumstances.

Some psychiatric drugs are more *teratogenic* (teratogenesis is a term used to indicate the development of abnormal structures in an embryo; the result is a severely deformed fetus) than others, especially LITHIUM (see page 276) and benzodiazepines (see pages 211–219). LITHIUM, for example, is a risky drug to use during the first trimester. If a medication is needed to treat a manic illness (for which LITHIUM normally would be the best choice for a nonpregnant woman), TEGRETOL (page 280) is the preferred drug. Instead of benzodiazepine sedatives, the pregnant woman might consider the use of antihistamines, such as ATARAX or VISTARIL (page 226). (See the chart on page 69 for FDA Categories of Drug Use During Pregnancy.)

Before using any drugs during a pregnancy, you should consult a physician. No one should ever abuse drugs, and especially not during a pregnancy. Alcohol abuse, for example, can lead to irreversible birth abnormalities, referred to as *fetal alcohol syndrome* (FAS). Other drugs should also be avoided, such as nicotine— since smoking, which adversely affects the fetal blood supply, can lead to low birth weight (LBW) babies. Of course, it is crucial that you abstain from any unauthorized use of opiates or narcotics whether pregnant or not.

FDA CATEGORIES OF DRUG USE DURING PREGNANCY

Category A: Reliable studies in pregnant women are negative [no significant risk] for fetal abnormalities.

Risk to fetus is remote.

Category B: Information from animal studies or reliable studies in pregnant women is negative [no significant risk].

Risk to fetus is relatively unlikely.

Category C: Either information from animal studies may be positive (significant risk) for fetal abnormalities or all reliable studies in pregnant women are not available.

Possible benefits of the drug are thought to warrant use despite potential risks to the fetus.

Category D: Studies in pregnant women or experience with the use of the drug has revealed evidence of fetal risk.

Only a serious or life-threatening situation warrants the use of this drug.

Category X: Evidence in animal studies, human pregnancy studies, or experience with the use of drug have proven positive (significant risk), for fetal abnormalities.

Use of this drug is contraindicated.

Breast-Feeding

Many psychiatric drugs taken by a lactating woman will show up in her milk. Sedatives, for example, may cross into the milk and affect not only the baby's sleep pattern but also the feeding pattern as well. However, the amount of the drug in the milk and its effect on the nursing infant will vary greatly, depending on the chemical characteristics of the drug, the dosage, and the duration of use.

The medications most likely to enter the breast milk are those that are most fat soluble, that is, drugs absorbed and stored in the mother's fat and passed into her milk in this form. Since drugs usually enter in small amounts, taking small doses of a drug for short periods is usually safer for the lactating mother than higher doses over long periods.

Again, the use of drugs during pregnancy or nursing period must be seen on a risk/benefit ratio: the potential health risks to the fetus or nursing child weighed against the possible benefits of the drug. If drugs are used during either period, the mother and child should be closely monitored by a physician. Of course, if drugs are necessary to the health of the nursing or lactating mother, bottle-feeding may be a viable alternative.

Children and Adolescents

The use of psychiatric medications for children and adolescents is controversial. The specific conditions for prescription drug use among children are less clear than among adults, and it is not always easy to separate variations in maturing behavior of young children, such as when they are *acting out* as opposed to what would be abnormal or aberrant behavior.

Psychiatric medicines are to be used carefully in children because they affect various systems and organs in the body. Consequently, physicians are reluctant to give most psychiatric medications to young developing children. However, some medications are thought to be relatively safe, and others may be prescribed if it is functionally necessary or life-saving. An example would be the use of certain types of antidepressants in a severely depressed adolescent.

From a physiological point of view, small children require lower doses of any medication because they clearly weigh less. Moreover, the difference in their body composition, fat deposition, the development of enzyme systems in the liver, and their ability to excrete from their kidneys (adult kidneys are far more efficient) are part of the complex relationships that determine what is an accurate dose for children.

If given psychiatric medication, children should receive the lowest effective dose and only of those drugs with documented safety for the specific age groups. For example, some psychiatric drugs are considered safe for children as young as two years, while other drugs are considered safe only for children twelve years and older. Again, a psychiatrist or your pediatrician will advise you as to the appropriate drug for your child.

Frequently, the same psychiatric conditions that develop in adults occur also in children: *schizophrenia,* which is a group of mental disorders characterized by disturbed thinking, mood, or behavior, and *Gilles de la Tourette's syndrome* are but two examples. In these instances, the same drugs used by adults are prescribed for children—except at greatly reduced levels.

Children are also given psychiatric medication for behavior or conduct disorders peculiar to them. The best example is attention-deficit disorder (ADD), often signalled by an inability to concentrate in school, which is usually accompanied by hyperactivity. The use of medication to treat this problem of constant restlessness, distractibility, and impulsiveness is controversial and requires the strictest diagnostic evaluation. But when satisfied that medication is an appropriate part of the therapy, the psychiatrist may have the choice of three types of medications: psychostimulants, such as RITALIN (page 240), certain tricyclic antidepressants, such as TOFRANIL (page 99), and LITHIUM (page 276).

Other problems for which psychiatric medications—namely the tricyclic antidepressant TOFRANIL—are used in children are sleeping difficulties. These kinds of problems range from bed-wetting to sleepwalking. Bed-wetting or *enuresis* can be a common problem in children six years and older, but it is not considered serious. Many parents successfully treat this problem by reducing the amount of liquid the child drinks before bedtime while increasing the amount of salt they eat by adding such snacks to their diet as potato chips or pretzels. The salt is beneficial since it encourages the retention of water in the body. If the problem persists, you should consult your pediatrician.

It should not be necessary to tell parents that medicating children with adult drugs is foolish and dangerous. However, I know of several instances in which a teething child was given a half-dose of VALIUM by his parents to help him sleep—as well as the parents. I do not know if this was a regular practice—I can only hope not—nor did I learn if the child suffered in any fashion. The fact is that any damage would not be known until many years later, if at all.

The use of psychiatric medication in children is becoming more refined as our body of information and study increases. But any use of medicines must be established on the basis of a firm evaluation and medical supervision so as not to alter the normal physical and psychological growth of children.

The Elderly

Although the elderly can be as sensitive as children or adolescents to the effects of certain psychiatric drugs, I believe the elderly are often not well supervised in their use of these medications. Therefore, I insist that someone in the household monitor the scheduled use of any psychiatric drugs taken by a senior member of the family and closely watch the patient for any side effects.

I find it helpful to tell both the elderly and other family members that as we all age the rate at which we metabolize our food and drugs slows down. Hence, drugs can accumulate in our body and their effects last longer. In some cases, toxicity may develop. Consequently, the elderly should receive only the lowest effective dosage of any psychiatric drug. And, for this reason, I tell everyone that increasing their dosage, no matter what the justification, is risky and unwarranted unless supervised by a doctor.

Whenever possible, the most suitable drugs for the elderly are short- rather than long-acting. Short-acting drugs, by definition, get in and out of the body relatively quickly. The long-acting drugs do not.

Drugs that have little likelihood of producing anticholingeric effects—such as blurred vision, constipation, increased heart rate, and possible mental confusion—are preferred. For example, when treating depression in the elderly, NORPRAMIN (page 103) is superior to ELAVIL (page 97) since NORPRAMIN produces fewer and less severe incidents of low blood pressure (hypotension) in the elderly and, therefore, reduces the possibility of an injury due to a fall.

The elderly often are medicated for multiple health problems. For example, many of the elderly are treated for hypertension, which is chronic high blood pressure. Yet many antihypertensive drugs, coupled with any one of several different types of psychiatric drugs, can sharply increase the risk of a potentially dangerous drug interaction. (See "Drug Interactions," page 20.)

As with children, family members should not take it upon themselves to medicate an elderly member of the family. The elderly react very sensitively to most psychiatric drugs. For example, someone aged seventy given VALIUM for less than one week because he or she was restless at night could easily experience toxic delirium, that is, he or she could become confused and disoriented. This reaction might happen even if the drug was discontinued after only five nights. Since their kidneys and liver often do not function well, the elderly do not effectively excrete the drugs. Consequently, they are always at risk of accumulating toxic levels of the drug in their body.

The elderly suffer from a greater risk of anticholinergic side effects of many antidepressants and antipsychotic medications, such as dry mouth and urinary retention. A medication intended to treat such side effects is an oral preparation, pilocarpine, whose brand name is SALAGEN.

Besides not sharing drugs with the elderly, if a senior member of your family is taking psychiatric drugs, notify the doctor promptly if you notice any unusual or adverse symptoms. The doctor will probably stop the drug immediately and observe the patient to learn if the symptoms are related to the drug or another ailment.

Other Health Factors That Affect
Drug Use

Ironically, a healthy person responds better to medication than a sick person. Drugs might not only further undermine someone's poor health, but the poor health can actually impair the effectiveness of the drug. Therefore, both your current health and health history are important items to share with your doctor before any psychiatric drug is prescribed. (See "What Your Doctor Needs to Know," page 18.) The following are only a small sample of those health issues that affect drug use.

Kidney and Liver Disease

Most drugs are broken down or metabolized in the liver and disposed of through the action of the kidneys. If someone suffered from any form of liver and kidney disease that caused those organs not to perform properly, such as people with advanced diabetes, drugs might accumulate in the body at alarmingly high levels. This condition might develop even if the drug had been administered at the normal levels. In these circumstances, the doctor might consider reducing the dosage and frequency of the medication to get the same effect.

Malabsorption

Oral drugs are, of course, absorbed through the stomach and intestine. Chronic inflammatory disorders that affect the small intestine, such as celiac disease or ileitis, produce symptoms that include chronic diarrhea and loss of appetite. These illnesses not only reduce our ability to absorb our food but our drugs as well. Other problems of malabsorption that might temporarily impair drug effectiveness include intestinal surgery, irritable bowel syndrome (IBS), diverticulosis or periodic diarrhea.

Alcoholism

Some alcoholics, who suffer withdrawal symptoms because of their addiction, go through a period of detoxification in a hospital or a private clinic before they begin their program of recovery. To help detoxify or clear the body of the alcohol and its toxic effects, drugs are often used. Some of these drugs hasten the detoxification process by accelerating the alcoholic's metabolism, which breaks down the alcohol and speeds its departure from the body.

Unfortunately, the drugs that accelerate metabolism will also reduce the bioavailability of other drugs—at least while the medication is being used. For example, if someone were being treated for his or her alcohol-related depression with a tricyclic antidepressant, the detoxifying medication would reduce that drug's effectiveness.

Blood Pressure
People who are receiving medication for their hypertension must check with their doctor to learn what drug interactions are possible when they begin to take a psychiatric drug. For example, if used in high doses, the combination of many antidepressants and monoamine-oxidase (MAO) inhibitors may cause severe excitation or seizures.

Hypotension
The effect of psychiatric drugs on blood pressure levels is an issue for another group of people, namely those people who have a very sensitive or *liable* nervous system for responding to changes in their blood pressure. Over the years, they have probably experienced moments of dizziness or suffered from various kinds of motion sickness. As children, they might have been carsick or, as adults, they feel queasy or their heart sinks when in an elevator. If these same people take various psychiatric drugs, they are more likely to experience orthostatic hypotension than others. That is, they may become dizzy more easily because they are especially sensitive or predisposed to the occasional drop in blood pressure these medicines cause.

Perspiration
A common side effect of many psychiatric drugs is sweating. People excessively sensitive to this problem have a very active

exocrine or secreting system. Called *secretors*, these people sweat a great deal even under normal conditions. If they take any of the tricyclic antidepressants, such as TOFRANIL, their sweating can become exaggerated. They are at no serious health risks associated with heavy sweating; however, the sweating prompted by the drug may be a great nuisance and possibly a cause of some noncompliance.

As I mentioned before, it is critical that before your doctor prescribes any psychiatric drug for you, he or she should have a full understanding of your health status and history. As to what is important to share about your medical history, I suggest you mention not only the health issues mentioned above, but any illness that required medical attention and especially medication.

FIVE

Drug Misuse and Abuse

Let me say that as an instrument of healing and recovery, drugs are to be used *only* when they are needed and, when no longer needed, they should be discontinued. A simple working definition of drug misuse or abuse is this: any use of a drug other than as prescribed by a doctor, including how, why, and when a drug is taken.

I make a personal and somewhat arbitrary distinction between two words: *misuse* and *abuse*. *Abuse*, as everyone knows, has been most widely accepted as the use of any illegal drug, such as heroin, LSD, or cocaine, especially because they have little or no therapeutic value. I also use the term to mean any *intentional* or knowing misuse of any prescription or nonprescription drug. On the other hand, I usually apply the term *misuse* to the unintentional, yet inappropriate, use of a prescription or nonprescription drug. I make a distinction between these two terms only because some of my patients who did not understand why and how they were misusing their drugs, did not want—nor deserved—to be labeled a *drug abuser*. For many of the same reasons, psychiatrists usually use the term *dependent* in place of *addictive* (see sidebar, page 83). However, I do not want to minimize the importance of wrongly using drugs. The misuse of a medication can easily lead to its abuse.

Misconceptions That Lead to Misuse

Understanding the habit-forming properties of specific psychiatric drugs is part of safe use practices for everyone. Unfortunately, a good number of the people I see do not know that many psychiatric drugs are habit-forming or *addicting*—even those drugs which some of them have already had a history of taking before seeing me. As with most health-care professionals, I agree that ignorance plays a major role in psychiatric drug-dependency problems. Studies reveal that a majority of people who initially became dependent upon psychiatric drugs did so unintentionally.

A common misunderstanding involves what to do when a dose is *missed*. In an effort to be faithful to a fixed drug regimen, people take double the prescribed amount when they have missed a single dose. The thinking is this: since my symptoms may return if I miss a dose, I can *catch up* by doubling up on the next dose.

The truth of the matter is that doubling the dose of a psychiatric medication, for whatever reason, usually increases the risk of an adverse reaction. It could also lead to a dangerous habit-forming practice if doses were missed frequently. If you happen to miss a dose, do not worry. Skip the missed dose and resume your normal drug regimen. Whatever symptoms, if any, that might appear due to the missed dosage will disappear as soon as you are back on your regular schedule.

Another mistaken belief is "more is better": people will *increase* their dosage when their symptoms are not relieved. If they become impatient with the latency period, people may increase the dosage within the first week—not realizing that it takes from one to two weeks before the drug will take effect. (See "Latency Period," page 35.) The fact is that psychiatric drugs need time to be effective; some may need as much as four to six weeks to reach their maximum effectiveness.

People also *increase* their dosage if they believe their symptoms have returned, especially after a number of weeks of drug use. If your drug begins to lose its effectiveness, it may be the sign of drug tolerance, which means it is time for you to see your doctor—but not the time for you to increase the amount of medication you take. (See "Tolerance," page 191.)

A quite opposite problem develops when symptoms diminish or disappear. On these occasions some people *decrease* their dosage. In some instances, they actually stop taking their medication altogether, and usually abruptly. Without a doctor's approval or supervision, the decrease or termination of a psychiatric drug can be a threat to your health. Frankly, if people stopped their medications as soon as their symptoms disappeared, the more likely response is that the symptoms would return—and possibly with greater intensity. (See "Terminating Psychiatric Medication," page 84.)

Perhaps the most insidious type of misuse involves indications: taking a drug for a purpose other than that indicated by the drug or doctor. A common practice of such misuse is referred to as *extended use* or *generalizing* its use. For instance, people receive tranquilizers from their medical doctor for the relief of anxiety symptoms prior to surgery. If they also decided to take the drug to reduce the anxiety or stress of day-to-day living, it would be considered *generalizing* its use. Even a decision to treat a seemingly quite legitimate problem of insomnia with a psychiatric drug should not be made without a doctor's supervision and not with a drug indicated for another purpose.

Generalizing your use of a drug is basically a bad policy because every treatable situation calls for, first, a specific diagnosis prior to recommending a treatment and medication. For example, tranquilizers are not all the same. One tranquilizer may be appropriate for one problem or person and totally inappropriate for another person. For example, DALMANE (page 211) and NOLUDAR (page 204) are both used to treat short-term insomnia but they are not precisely the same drugs. The former is far more risky for a pregnant woman and the latter causes an incidence of increased dreaming or nightmares when it is stopped. And neither one of them should be used over an extended period of time.

Consequently, do not make your own medical decisions by

extending or generalizing the use of one of your drugs. Take your medications only for what they are prescribed—and no more. This is not only the safest policy, but the best medicine.

Dependence Liability

Dependence liability means a drug has a quality which by its use might reenforce its reuse. More specifically, the drug stimulates an aspect of the reward center of the central nervous system which causes a pleasant sensation—sometimes intense, sometimes not. For some people, the sensation is sufficiently impelling for them to continue the drug's use beyond any therapeutic value. Other people become so dependent on the genuine therapeutic effect of the drug that life without it seems unbearable. An example would be chronic insomniacs for whom a night's sleep is impossible without medication.

It does not follow that merely using dependent-liable drugs will produce drug-dependent habits. Frankly, drug dependency is still statistically very uncommon among the millions of people who use psychiatric drugs. But for the people who use a highly dependent-liable medication for an extended period, a *biological adaptation* occurs. Basically, the cells of the brain become so accustomed or adapted to the presence of the drug that a sort of reliance develops; when the drug is withdrawn, the cells object to the sense of deprivation they feel.

As explained earlier in the section on latency periods, the cells of our brain need a week or two to become accustomed or adapted to the presence of a psychiatric drug. However, with most dependent-liable drugs, a tolerance also begins to develop. This means that if the drug is maintained at the same dosage level, it eventually begins to become less effective. Consequently, for the drug to maintain the same level of effectiveness, it is necessary to increase the dosage of the drug.

Also, when the drug becomes such an intrinsic part of the

workings of the brain cells, any sudden decrease or absence of the drug leads to a characteristic response known as an *abstinence syndrome* or *withdrawal symptoms*. In effect, the brain cells object to the loss of a substance they have come to accept as natural and necessary.

Needless to say, all dependent-liable medications should be dispensed only under close medical supervision. These drugs also should never be terminated unilaterally or abruptly.

DANGER SIGNS OF DRUG DEPENDENCY

The following are some of the more common signs of a potential, if not actual, drug dependency.

1. Unexpected persistence or worsening of symptoms, such as anxiety or pain, despite what seems to be normal recovery time following use of the drug.
2. The illness for which the symptom was originally treated exceeds the expected time of recovery.
3. Increased dosage by the patient without medical supervision. (Evidence of a physiological or psychological adaptation of the drug to the cells of the central nervous system that makes incremental increases of the drug necessary to get the same results.)
4. Use of the drug for heretofore normal activities of daily living, such as getting up in the morning or going to bed.
5. Irritability or defensiveness when the drug user is confronted about his or her use.
6. Sudden mood changes, irritability, accident-proneness, clumsiness, deterioration of personal habits, lateness or absences at work.
7. When upward changes in the dosage of the drug lead to a state of hyperactivity in the central nervous system: hyperalertness, muscle cramps, anxiety, restlessness and, in the worse case, seizures (further evidence of the obligatory nature of the drug's presence in the body's central nervous system).
8. Failed attempts, perhaps repeated failures, at stopping the drug.

Qualities of Dependent-Liable Medications

The basic quality that makes drugs dependent-liable is that they can directly or indirectly stimulate the naturally occurring reward system of our bodies. In the course of our lives, we appropriately experience pleasure, that is, physical and psychological stimulation and satisfaction in many different circumstances: two examples would be food and sex. Certain drugs can elicit similar but far more intense feelings by stimulating this reward system. Consequently, some people will consistently and persistently take these drugs only for the sake of their pleasure-producing qualities, even at the expense of their more vital functions, such as eating or drinking—or sex.

The drugs that are most abused or abusable are those that are rapid- or short-acting. In a very short period of time, the drug enters the body, crosses the blood-brain barrier, and enters the brain in large concentrations. In the same fashion, they exit the body quickly. Because these drugs break down or metabolize rapidly, they also dissipate quickly. This rapid onset of action and decay has an equally swift effect on someone's moods—a so-called *saw-tooth effect*. It causes a rapid change of mood from neutral to euphoria; then, as the drug decays, it moves to dysphoria or exaggerated depression. This cycle of euphoria and dysphoria is what leads to reuse of the drug as the user wants to both reestablish the euphoria and get rid of the dysphoria. In principle, this is the dynamic a crack addict faces: intense euphoria ("it's like falling in love") and equally potent depression and anguish.

It was not so long ago that our profession did not fully appreciate the potency of some dependent-liable drugs. For example, benzodiazepines are widely used in this country in the treatment of anxiety and insomnia. They also carry with them a dependence-liability; namely, they can be addictive.

For years these same benzodiazepines were thought to be suitable drugs for treating alcohol-withdrawal symptoms and alleviating the anxiety that may have prompted the alcohol abuse. Unfortunately, many recovering patients, while eased from the use of alcohol, would find themselves (weeks later) dependent on benzodiazepines. Until the problem of dependency was discovered in those people treated with the benzodiazepines, alcoholics with symptoms of anxiety were frequently prescribed VALIUM, an antianxiety benzodiazepine. Although VALIUM is no longer recommended in these circumstances, even today some practitioners still use several of the less potent benzodiazepines, such as TRANXENE (page 255), because they are effective. But, by and large, the preferred drugs in the treatment of drug-withdrawal symptoms are nonbenzodiazepine medications, such as the antiseizure agent TEGRETOL (page 280).

Another class of drugs with dependence-liabilities is hypnotic sedatives, such as PLACYDYL (page 205) and DORIDEN (page 207), two drugs prescribed for short-term insomnia. Because of their known *addictive* qualities, these two drugs should generally not be used for much more than seven days—consecutively.

Finally, psychostimulants, such as DEXEDRINE, RITALIN, and PONDIMIN (page 243), are also habit-forming because of their dependent qualities. For these reasons, I discourage people from using these drugs over any extended period and definitely not as an appetite depressant.

DEPENDENT VERSUS ADDICTIVE

Technically, the term *addiction* is no longer used. The more generic, albeit ambiguous, term is *dependency*. The reason for the change is primarily a matter of stigmatism: the addict (and addiction) had wrongly come to be seen as someone who resorted to criminal activities in order to satisfy his or her need for illegal drugs. The dark associations with the word made it difficult to deal with people's fears about the potential addictive or dependency effects of many psychiatric drugs. Moreover, their lingering fears of becoming addicted caused people to either reduce the dosages of their medications or stop taking them altogether. In some cases, people refused to take certain psychiatric drugs because of their addictive *reputation*.

Changing a word may not deter someone from misusing a drug if they so choose; but it may make it easier to talk more candidly about the limits of drug use without unnecessarily alarming people with language that has unlawful associations.

Terminating Psychiatric Medication

After effectively using a psychiatric drug for a couple of months or more to eliminate specific symptoms, if you do not properly discontinue the drug, all your good work can be lost. Much as mountain climbers claim that coming down is more treacherous than climbing up, terminating a drug requires more care than starting it.

Unfortunately, the improper cessation of medication may be one of the most common of all causes for a recurrence of psychiatric illnesses or disorders. As evidence of this problem, large numbers of the psychiatric inpatient admissions in many psychiatric hospitals are associated with a recurrence of symptoms due to a failure to comply with drug regimens.

When stopping drugs with high tolerance qualities, such as benzodiazepines, you need to slowly reduce your dosage over time—as much as two weeks. To suddenly stop taking these medications is to risk a variety of withdrawal or *rebound* symptoms— such as anxiety, sleeplessness, or depression—that may last as long as seventy-two hours to a week. Abrupt discontinuation of a major tranquilizer, such as THORAZINE, can also cause highly dramatic symptoms, such as tremors and other abnormal, involuntary movements. (See "Dyskinesia," page 289.)

When rebound symptoms occur, people may view the event as confirming evidence that their medication is not effective or, worse, that they have become *addicted* to the drug.

Your policy should be that if you have used a psychiatric drug for many months, whether it is considered highly dependent-forming or not, do not stop its use abruptly. This practice is true of almost any drug you use to alter your mood, even that non-prescription antihistamine that helps you fall asleep at night.

Over time, your body makes both biological and psychological adjustments to the presence of a drug in your system. If a change is made in the drug's status, such as your taking less of it or stopping it altogether, you may experience an unwanted reaction. For example, many people routinely take aspirin every night in order to sleep better, even though pharmacologically aspirin has no sedating qualities. But once the aspirin routine is established, it takes on hypnotic qualities for people. This placebo effect (page 36) is a perfectly legitimate use of the medication, as long as it is used in moderation. What many of these people discover is that if they terminate the aspirin use abruptly, their insomnia returns. The abrupt withdrawal of the drug leads to something called *symptom breakthrough*, which is a return of the symptoms for which you had been taking the drug in the first place. In this case, more sleepless nights. On the other hand, to avoid this kind of problem, you should gradually reduce the dosage and frequency of aspirin use for about a week. (Regular aspirin use is an issue you should discuss with your physician.)

In addition to aspirin, other over-the-counter drugs can also produce so-called *functional addictions*. For example, if your body has come to depend upon a laxative for regularity, the constipation may be made worse if you discontinue its use—and certainly if you stop abruptly. Nasal sprays are another example: people who have abused the use of the nasal sprays found that when they stopped using them, their nose became stuffed sooner and they felt even worse.

So, once again, if you take any medication over time that can potentially produce a functional dependence, consider tapering off its use before stopping completely. It's a prudent policy; it may also save you some anxious moments. In Chapter 6, "Psychiatric Drug Profiles," you will find more specific advice on those drugs which require careful tapering procedures before finally being discontinued.

IMPORTANT FACTORS FOR TAPERING DEPENDENT-LIABLE DRUGS

1. You feel ready and confident to terminate your medication.
2. Your doctor has told you the length of the tapering period and the planned schedule for gradually reducing the dosage.
3. You are symptom-free and functioning as well as you had before the symptoms first appeared.
4. You are no longer preoccupied with anxiety.
5. You are not entering into your premenstrual cycle.
6. You do not foresee any additional sources of stress during the tapering period.

Washout Period

As we have discussed, the majority of psychiatric medications should be tapered over a period of time before they are completely stopped. The body and psyche need time to readjust to the absence of the drug. In addition to those drugs for which you need to taper their use to avoid withdrawal symptoms, some drugs require a further period of time, called a *washout* period, before the body is free of any lingering traces of the drug. These long-lasting drugs leave the body slowly.

A washout period is important to observe since you cannot begin to take any number of other drugs until your body is completely purged of the previous drug. More specifically, during a washout period, you may not take any other drug of the same family or a drug that could possibly cause an adverse reaction. If you make a drug substitution during this washout period, you run the risk of serious adverse effects. If your doctor found it necessary to change your medication, in some instances there are drugs of another family that can be used as a temporary substitute.

A washout period lasts anywhere from seven to fourteen days, depending upon the drug. A drug such as PROZAC requires at least a week's washout, and others, such as monoamine-oxidase

(MAO) inhibitors, need at least a full two weeks before another drug can be safely taken.

I recently faced a situation that illustrates the need for an appropriate washout period. It concerned a man who had been taking MAO inhibitors for depression. He had to stop the drug because of the dietary restrictions associated with their use. (See "Tyramine-Rich Foods," page 88.) Within three days he had switched to NORPRAMIN (page 103), a tricyclic antidepressant. By the second day on this new drug he had an intense headache and his nose bled—signs of dangerously high blood pressure. When he called and told me what the situation was, I told him to stop the NORPRAMIN. Those symptoms suggested his hypertension was so severe that, if he had taken the drug much longer, he could have suffered a stroke or worse. Once he stopped the medication, however, his blood pressure returned to normal levels and his symptoms disappeared.

The irony was that this man had dropped the MAO inhibitors because he did not want to accept the constraints on his diet. The food restrictions were necessary in order to protect him from a very specific food-and-drug interaction that occurs with that drug and tyramine-rich foods: high blood pressure.

In summary, always follow your doctor's instructions when stopping psychiatric drugs, especially those with high dependence liabilities. If for any reason any of your original symptoms reappear during the tapering period, your doctor can make small adjustments, such as slowing down the tapering process or prolonging it. And follow your doctor's advice regarding any dietary restrictions involving the use of MAO inhibitors.

Signs of Drug Dependency

In addition to learning those side effects that are common to the drug you are using, take time to discover what effects or reactions would be clear indications that you should stop taking the drug—and see your doctor.

TYRAMINE-RICH FOODS

Monoamine-oxidase (MAO) inhibitors block the action of an enzyme called the monoamine-oxidase enzyme. This means the effectiveness of the drug is linked to making the enzyme ineffective. However, among other tasks, the enzyme is needed to destroy a food substance called tyramine that is found in a variety of foods we commonly eat. This food substance normally is converted in the body to an inactive form by the enzyme. But when, for example, MAO inhibitors suppress the level of the enzyme, the tyramine remains active. This causes a problem. The active tyramine produces a release of the neurotransmitter norepinephrine, which is a brain chemical that prompts the blood vessels to constrict. When the blood vessels compress, it produces a sharp, even dangerous rise in blood pressure.

Tyramine is found in a variety of foods, especially aged cheeses and pickled food. The following are common foods known to be rich in tyramine:

alcoholic beverages (e.g., beer, Chianti, and sherry)
bananas
bologna
cheeses (e.g., boursault, Brie, Camembert, cheddar, Gruyère, Parmesan, Romano, Roquefort, and Stilton)
chocolate
eggplant
hot dogs
liver
pepperoni
pineapple
plums
salami
soy sauce

There is a dynamic relationship between some of the food we eat and the drugs we take that requires us to respect the dietary restrictions prescribed along certain drugs—especially MAO inhibitors. Safe use of these particular drugs is definitely linked to the avoidance of tyramine-containing foods.

The first thing to understand about signs of drug dependency is that they are not always obvious. But they are to be taken seriously in that they all lead to grave and, sometimes, life-threatening situations.

Adverse symptoms are often dose-related: the more you take of the drug, the more likely you will experience those symptoms. They may also occur if you take a larger dose or take the drug more frequently than was prescribed. In effect, they may be indications of drug abuse.

The signs of an overdose or drug abuse are not always easily recognized. Symptoms will vary from drug to drug and person to person. However, people who gradually develop a drug dependency usually exhibit specific changes in their behavior that gradually show up in their work performance or personal relationships. The kind of behavior I mean is frequently erratic. The drug causes unpredictable mood changes, usually alternating between (1) *periods of exhilaration and agitation* with (2) *intervals of exhaustion and lethargy.*

Yet all signs of drug dependency are not so dramatic. An early indication may be either insomnia or a need to sleep for long periods of time, often referred to as *crashing.* Some people lose interest in eating or have to drink inordinate amounts of water to satiate their thirst. Bloodshot eyes or eyes that have a dazed or expressionless appearance can also suggest drug abuse. Even excessive sweating or flushed skin, or an unexplained rash may be a sign.

So, pay attention to what you are doing when taking a psychiatric drug. Follow your doctor's instructions and report any persistent or disruptive symptoms. But even if you have not experienced any troubling symptoms, if you are not following the prescriptive instructions of your doctor, you are still abusing the drug. If you continue to change your drug schedule, time will tell: the symptoms of abuse will appear and the longer you abuse a drug, the more likely they will be severe.

SIX

Psychiatric Drug Profiles

Antidepressant drugs were introduced in this country in the early 1960s. The largest category of antidepressants is called *tricyclic* (TCA), a name that refers to the nature of their chemical structure. These drugs affect the symptoms of depression by adjusting how the brain and nervous system produces and responds to their own natural chemicals, called neurotransmitters (such as norepinephrine, serotonin, and dopamine).

Most psychiatrists will select tricyclic antidepressants as their first choice of drugs in treating long-term depression; on the other hand, they should not be used to treat the symptoms of short-term or transitory depression.

In addition to lifting depression and elevating mood, these drugs can improve sleep, increase physical activity and mental alertness, improve appetite, and generally restore interest in everyday life. Some doctors will also use certain tricyclic antidepressants to control chronic pain, prevent the onset of migraine, treat pathological weeping, sleep apnea, peptic ulcer disease, and attention-deficit disorder.

Course of Treatment

Antidepressants are to be taken in multi-dose regimens, that is, several doses each day, usually at the beginning of a drug treatment program. Once the level of necessary medication has been established, some antidepressants can be taken in single doses, usually at night, a practice called *night-loading*. These drugs will begin to reduce depression only after two weeks of use; the actual course of treatment may range from three weeks to three months. If the problem is recurrent depression, the therapy may involve long-term or *maintenance* use (perhaps years) of a low-dose drug.

The treatment of depressive symptoms with these types of medication usually unfolds in these stages:

1. Within a few days or the first week of treatment, the medication should diminish or eliminate any anxiety symptoms associated with the depression.
2. Within two or three weeks, symptoms of chronic fatigue and lack of energy should be eased or eliminated, and a natural sleep pattern should be restored.
3. Mood elevation and sexual function, usually the last to return, may take up to four weeks after the initiation of antidepressants.

Note: All progress should be routinely discussed with your doctor.

Potential Risks

As with all psychiatric drug use, there is some risk of side effects and, less so, of adverse reactions. However, some people are at greater risk than others.

Children   Because this group of drugs can pose a risk for children, most of them are not recommended for patients under twelve, and the drug ASENDIN should not be given to anyone under the age of sixteen. One exception is the drug TOFRANIL, which can be given safely to children as young as six years in the treatment of bed-wetting (enuresis). In every instance of drug use, the weight, general health, and severity of the symptoms of the child should be taken into consideration before any antidepressant medication is prescribed.

Women   The safety of all antidepressant drugs for use during pregnancy has not been established. The growing tissues of the fetus are extremely sensitive to the presence of foreign chemicals such as drugs, especially during the early periods of life. Hence, it is important that you speak to your physician before using any antidepressant drugs during pregnancy. However, depending upon the particular antidepressant drug, it is thought that some (if not all) of them can be used *if the need is clear* and *the potential benefits to the mother outweigh the potential risks to the fetus*. For your help, at the close of each drug entry is a specific category of risk for its use during pregnancy.

Also, if you intend to breast-feed, consult with your doctor since tricyclic antidepressants appear in breast milk. (For more information about the use of drugs during pregnancy, see "Pregnant and Lactating Women," page 66.)

Elderly   Low doses of these drugs are usually safer and sufficient for most elderly. The principal health risk associated with these drugs for people over the age of sixty is the potential for developing heart rhythm abnormalities. (See "The Elderly," page 72.)

In those medications where an adverse risk of tardive dyskinesia is present, especially among antipsychotic drugs, such as PROLIXIN, MOBAN, and COMPAZINE, it is thought that people of Asian ancestry are at greater risk than African Americans, with whites at the lowest risk.

Withdrawal

If these drugs are abruptly stopped after long-term use or high-dose therapy, you may experience symptoms such as dizziness, headaches, nausea, depression, and nightmares. These symptoms may begin within two to four days and last as long as two weeks.

Even if you taper off or gradually reduce the use of the drug, you may experience a little irritability, sleeplessness, or nervousness for a few days. Consequently, your doctor can tell you, specifically, how to come off a particular drug with the fewest side effects. (For more advice about discontinuing psychiatric drugs, see "Terminating Psychiatric Medication," page 84.)

Food-and-Drug Interactions
If your urine is not sufficiently acidic (that is to say, if it is too alkaline), it can prolong the effect of these drugs in your body. Usually, your diet will not have a significant effect on the alkalinity of your urine, unless of course it consists almost exclusively of alkaline-producing foods, such as dairy products and vegetables (excluding corn and lentils). For the same reasons, you should also avoid antacids that neutralize stomach acid while taking these drugs, because by reducing the acid they will make your urine more alkaline. Alcohol should not be consumed while taking these drugs because it can increase intoxication and possibly induce depression. If you feel the need to drink even small quantities of alcohol while taking antidepressants, it is best to consult your doctor first.

Those individuals consuming a high-fiber diet must understand that it can interfere with all absorption and, therefore, increase the blood levels of tricyclic antidepressants.

Side Effects
Side effects occur for a variety of reasons. Their frequency and severity depend on factors such as the strength of the dose, how long someone has taken the drug, and, of course, the susceptibility of the user. (See "People at Particular Risk," page 66.) For example, antidepressant drugs may trigger an episode of mania in people predisposed to or known to have suffered from bipolar depression (see page 288). These side effects are more likely to occur in SSRIs and MAO-inhibitor medications than tricyclic antidepressant drugs.

Physiological Effects of Antidepressants

Behavioral   Excitement; anxiety; nervousness; panic; insomnia; confusion; memory loss.

Blood system   Abnormal blood count and blood-sugar tests.

Circulatory system   Heart palpitations; rapid pulse; orthostatic hypotension (dizziness when standing or changing position suddenly); increased blood pressure; abnormal heart rhythms.

Dermatological   Rash; itching and red or dry skin; hives; unusual bleeding or bruising; sensitivity to sunlight; hair loss; flushing; sweating; yellowing of the eyes (jaundice).

Digestive system   Nausea; vomiting, constipation; loss or increase in appetite; constipation; diarrhea; stomach cramps; rectal gas; difficulty swallowing.

Head and eyes   Blurred vision; glaucoma; dilated (wide) pupils; facial swelling; black tongue; nasal congestion.

Liver   Yellowing of the skin or eyes (jaundice); abnormal liver-function tests.

Nervous system   Headaches; fatigue; poor coordination; poor concentration.

Urinary and reproductive system   Swelling of the testicles; changes in sex drive; painful or difficult urination; irregular menstrual cycles; changes in breast milk production.

Other   Chills and fevers; male breast enlargement; changes in taste; changes in weight.

Guidelines for Use

In evaluating patients, a previous history of their use of antidepressants and their effectiveness, a history of the effectiveness of an antidepressant in a family member, and the history of side effects (if the patient has had a previous history with antidepressants) are important in determining the use and choice of antidepressants.

You will not feel the full effectiveness of these drugs for about two weeks, perhaps three. Hence, take the medication as prescribed: do not increase the dosage. A common side effect is drowsiness; avoid the use of other medicines, such as over-the-counter (OTC) cold medicine, or alcohol beverages, since they

may increase the drowsiness. Also, use extreme caution while
driving or using machinery that requires alertness or good coordination.

Always call your doctor if the drug causes any side effects that
persist for more than a week. Do not hesitate to notify your doctor
if you experience increased heartbeat, poor coordination, painful
or difficult urination, excessive drowsiness, impaired vision, or
sore throat and fever. If you experience constipation, take a stool
softener and increase your fluids.

ANTIDEPRESSANTS

FIRST-GENERATION TRICYCLICS

Brand Name	Generic Name
ELAVIL, ENDEP, EMITRIP, AMITRIL	amitriptyline (a-mee-TRIP-ti-leen)
TOFRANIL, TOFRANIL-PM, JANIMINE, TIPRAMINE	imipramine (im-IP-ra-meen)

SECOND-GENERATION TRICYCLICS

Brand Name	Generic Name
NORPRAMIN, PERTOFRANE	desipramine (dess-IP-ra-meen)
PAMELOR, AVENTYL	nortriptyline (nor-TRIP-ti-leen)
VIVACTIL, NEOACTIL	protriptyline (pro-TRIP-ti-leen)
SURMONTIL	trimipramine (trye-MIP-ra-meen)
ASENDIN	amoxapine (a-MOX-a-peen)
SINEQUAN, ADAPIN	doxepin (DOX-e-pin)
WELLBUTRIN	bupropion HCl (boo-PRO-pi-un)

SEROTONIN REUPTAKE BLOCKERS

Brand Name	Generic Name
DESYREL	trazodone (TRAZ-o-done)
PROZAC	fluoxetine (floo-OX-i-teen)
ANAFRANIL	clomipramine (klo-MIP-ra-meen)
LUVOX	fluvoxamine (floo-VOX-a-meen)
LUDIOMIL	maprotiline (ma-PRO-ti-leen)
EFFEXOR	venlafaxine (ven-la-FAX-een)
ZOLOFT	sertraline (SER-tra-leen)
PAXIL	paroxetine (pair-o-SET-een)
SERZONE	nefazadone (ne-FAZ-a-doan)

MONOAMINE-OXIDASE INHIBITORS

Brand Name	Generic Name
NARDIL	phenelzine (FEN-el-zeen)
MARPLAN	isocarboxazid (eye-so-kar-BOX-a-zid)
PARNATE	tranylcypromine (tran-ill-SIP-ro-meen)
EUTONYL	pargyline (PAR-gi-leen)
ELDEPRYL	selegiline (sell-e-GILL-een)

AUGMENTATION

Brand Name	Generic Name
LIMBITROL, LIMBITROL-DS	chlordiazepoxide (klor-dye-az-e-POX-ide) and amitriptyline (a-mee-TRIP-ti-leen)

THYROID HORMONE
LITHIUM
PSYCHOSTIMULANTS

FIRST-GENERATION TRICYCLICS

Brand Name
ELAVIL, ENDEP,
  EMITRIP, AMITRIL

Generic Name
amitriptyline (a-mee-
  TRIP-ti-leen)

HOW THE DRUG WORKS

By increasing the amount of norepinephrine or serotonin, or both, in the central nervous system, it improves nerve transmission.

PURPOSE

Fights depression, especially organic depression.

DOSAGE

Treatment of depression
Adults: (initially) 75 mg (taken orally) daily in divided doses, followed by an increase in the late-afternoon or bedtime dose, up to a maximum of 150 mg daily in divided doses; as an option, start with 50 mg to 100 mg at bedtime and, if needed, increase to 25 mg to 50 mg in the bedtime dose to a maximum of 150 mg daily in divided doses.

Adolescents and Elderly: (initially) 30 to 40 mg daily in divided doses; they should not be given more than 100 mg per day since they require less of the drug.

SIDE EFFECTS

Common: Dizziness; drowsiness; dry mouth; excessive sweating; weight gain; fatigue.
Uncommon: Constipation; diarrhea; vomiting.

ADVERSE REACTIONS

Blurred vision; skin rash; decreased sexual ability; anxiety; restlessness; eye pain; urinary retention; breast enlargement (in male); galactorrhea; trembling; unsteadiness; rapid heart beat; insomnia; nightmares.

DRUG INTERACTION

Increases the effects of drugs such as alcohol and other CNS depressants; narcotic analgesics; amphetaminelike drugs; atropine; oral anticoagulants.
Decreases the effects of clonidine and other antidepressant drugs.
With barbiturates, the effectiveness of the drug decreases.

With MAO inhibitors, fevers, delirium, severe excitation, or seizures may occur.

With epinephrine or norepinephrine, an increase in blood pressure may occur.

OVERDOSAGE

If any of the following symptoms develops, notify your physician immediately: Drowsiness; cold skin; congestive heart failure; fever; hallucinations; shortness of breath; muscle rigidity; vomiting.

Comments: Amitriptyline, developed in the 1960s, is the drug favored by many older, more experienced physicians because they are familiar with the drug, especially its side effects, and more confident of its general effectiveness. Since it is an excellent sedative, this drug is often given to people with sleeping difficulties in a single dose at night. People report improved sleep almost immediately, even before the depression has been relieved. This drug is also used to prevent the onset of cluster and migraine headaches, and to treat pathologic weeping and laughing associated with multiple sclerosis. Because it can be used to treat chronic pain, it is frequently prescribed by primary physicians, internists, and gynecologists. In some research centers, doctor have used 15 mg of ELAVIL daily to treat stubborn urinary-tract infections.

Yet, by today's standards, it is considered somewhat crude (as is imipramine, see below) since it affects more than one central nervous system and produces perhaps the widest range of anticholinergic side effects, such as drying of the mucus membrane, dry mouth, blurred vision, dizziness, constipation, and urinary hesitancies, of the tricyclic drug family. For this reason, the elderly should receive minimum dosages. Megadoses of vitamin C may reduce the effect of ELAVIL, as might heavy tobacco use.

This drug will produce few, if any, intended effects for the first two weeks of use, and full effect may take a month. When preparing to discontinue its use, do not stop abruptly: this can result in withdrawal symptoms such as irritability, restlessness, nightmares, and insomnia. If you experience constipation, increase your fluids; and if it persists, ask your doctor about a stool softener or laxative. This drug has been known to produce significant weight gain in some patients. If you have dry mouth, sugarless hard candy or chewing gum should bring adequate relief. Avoid drinking any alcohol whatsoever, as this drug can significantly increase both the intoxicating effects of alcohol and the ability of alcohol to cause depression.

Pregnancy: Category D (see sidebar on page 69). This means that studies in pregnant women have shown a positive risk to the fetus. Therefore, the drug should be used only if needed in a serious disease and when other safer drugs have proven to be ineffective or cannot be used.

Brand Name	*Generic Name*
TOFRANIL, TOFRANIL-PM, JANIMINE, TIPRAMINE	imipramine (im-IP-ra-meen)

HOW THE DRUG WORKS

By increasing the amount of norepinephrine or serotonin, or both, in the central nervous system, it improves nerve transmission.

PURPOSE

Depression, especially of a biological origin; sleep disorders; childhood enuresis (bed-wetting).

DOSAGE

Treatment of depression and sleep disorders
TOFRANIL

Adults: (initially) 75 mg (taken orally) daily in divided doses, morning and night; if necessary, your late-afternoon or evening dosages can be increased but your total daily divided doses should not exceed 150 mg/day *for outpatients*; usual maintenance dosage is 50 mg to 150 mg daily. *For hospitalized patients*, initial dosage is often 100 mg daily, followed by increases as needed; if no response is reached by the second week, increase the dosage to 250 mg or 300 mg daily.

Adolescents and Elderly: (initially) 30 mg to 40 mg daily, in divided doses; these people should not be given more than 100 mg per day since they require less of the drug.

Treatment of depression
TOFRANIL-PM

Adults: (initially) 75 mg (taken orally) daily in divided doses, followed by 150 mg daily and then 200 mg daily in divided doses *for outpatients*; after about three weeks, this drug can be taken at bedtime (the letters PM refer to bedtime use).

Treatment of enuresis

Children (over the age of six years): (initially) 25 mg daily, one hour before bedtime; if no satisfactory response is not reached after one week, increase dosage to 50 mg daily *in children under twelve* and 75 mg daily *in children over twelve*. For enuresis early in the night, give in divided doses: 25 mg mid-afternoon and 25 mg at bedtime.

SIDE EFFECTS

Common: Dizziness; drowsiness; dry mouth; excessive sweating; weight gain; fatigue.

Uncommon: Constipation; diarrhea; vomiting.

ADVERSE REACTIONS

Blurred vision; skin rash; decreased sexual ability; anxiety; restlessness; eye pain; urinary retention; breast enlargement (in male); galactorrhea; trembling; unsteadiness; rapid heart beat; insomnia; nightmares.

DRUG INTERACTION

Increases the effects of drugs such as alcohol and other CNS depressants; narcotic analgesics; amphetaminelike drugs; atropine; oral anticoagulants.
Decreases the effects of clonidine and other antidepressant drugs.

With barbiturates, the effectiveness of the drug decreases.
With MAO inhibitors, fevers, delirium, severe excitation, seizures, or death may occur.

With epinephrine or norepinephrine, an increase in blood pressure may occur.

OVERDOSAGE

If any of the following symptoms develops, notify your physician immediately: Drowsiness; cold skin; congestive heart failure; fever; hallucinations; shortness of breath; muscle rigidity; vomiting.

Comments: Another first-generation tricyclic antidepressant, the side effects of imipramine are much like those of amitriptyline, but less sedating. Hence, it is less likely to be used for depressed individuals who are also agitated. Rather, the drug is preferred for those people with *anergic depression*—a depression that leaves people listless, sluggish, and inactive. It should not be prescribed for insomnia as it can aggravate sleep problems, especially if taken in the evening. A better drug for insomnia is ELAVIL or ENDEP.

Occasionally doctors will prescribe TOFRANIL to control chronic pain. In addition, it is effective in treating a wide array of phobic conditions, such as agoraphobia (fear of open spaces) and, to a lesser degree, obsessive-compulsive disorders (OCD). It is also effective as a treatment for childhood enuresis (bed-wetting), although the mechanism of its action is still controversial.

Like ELAVIL or ENDEP, TOFRANIL produces a considerable number of typical anticholinergic side effects, such as drying of the mucus membrane, dry mouth, blurred vision, dizziness, constipation, and urinary hesitancies. The drug also has an impact on heart rhythm; all cardiac patients and their physicians must be aware of this side effect, especially when the drug is used among the elderly.

In some people, the use of the drug leads to appreciable weight gain, and its sedating qualities make it important for you to drive a car or operate machinery only when necessary. Alertness and motor coordination are affected by the drug.

The full effect of the drug will take from one to three weeks. When preparing to discontinue its use, do not stop abruptly: this can cause withdrawal symptoms, such as irritability, restlessness, nausea, and malaise. If you experience constipation, increase your fluids; and if it persists, ask your doctor about a stool softener or laxative. If you have dry mouth, sugarless hard candy or chewing gum should bring adequate relief. Avoid drinking alcohol completely; this drug can significantly increase both the intoxicating effects of alcohol and the ability of alcohol to cause depression.

Pregnancy: Category D (see sidebar on page 69). Studies in pregnant women have shown a significant risk to the fetus. Therefore, the drug should be used only if needed in a serious disease and when other, safer drugs have proven to be ineffective or cannot be used.

SECOND-GENERATION TRICYCLICS

The next group of antidepressant drugs, introduced in the early 1970s, was developed to make specific improvements on the amitriptyline and imipramine drugs: a shorter latency period (faster-acting); fewer side effects, particularly the acetylcholinergic side effects, such as low blood pressure, which are considerably troubling to the elderly; and a drug that would permit the doctor to tell objectively if the patient was getting an adequate amount of medicine. The latter virtue permits the doctor to draw a sample of blood and, through a simple chemical analysis, determine objectively whether your body is getting enough of the medication. This is sometimes called a *therapeutic window*.

Though it was hoped that these newer antidepressants would

be more rapid-acting and have more benign side effects than the earlier generation of drugs, only the latter benefit has been realized. The latency period of these new drugs—the time it takes for the drug to take effect—turned out to be the same as the first generation.

Brand Name	*Generic Name*
NORPRAMIN, PERTOFRANE	desipramine (dess-IP-ra-meen)

HOW THE DRUG WORKS

By increasing the amount of norepinephrine or serotonin, or both, in the central nervous system, it improves nerve transmission.

PURPOSE

Depression, especially of a biological origin.

DOSAGE

Treatment of depression
Adults: 100 mg to 200 mg (taken orally) daily in divided doses; for more severe depression, increase gradually, up to 300 mg daily.

SIDE EFFECTS

Common: Dizziness; drowsiness; dry mouth; excessive sweating; weight gain; fatigue.
Uncommon: Constipation; diarrhea; vomiting.

ADVERSE REACTIONS

Blurred vision; skin rash; decreased sexual ability; anxiety; restlessness; eye pain; urinary retention; breast enlargement (in male); galactorrhea; trembling; unsteadiness; rapid heart beat; insomnia; nightmares.

DRUG INTERACTION

Increases the effects of drugs such as alcohol and other CNS depressants; narcotic analgesics; amphetaminelike drugs; atropine; oral anticoagulants.

Decreases the effects of clonidine and other antidepressant drugs.

With barbiturates, the effectiveness of the drug decreases.

With MAO inhibitors, fevers, delirium, severe excitation, seizures, or death may occur.

With epinephrine or norepinephrine, an increase in blood pressure may occur.

OVERDOSAGE

If any of the following symptoms develops, notify your physician immediately: Drowsiness; cold skin; congestive heart failure; fever; hallucinations; shortness of breath; muscle rigidity; vomiting.

Comments: This second-generation antidepressant is a *metabolite* (or derivative) of imipramine. Its major asset is that it produces fewer anticholinergic effects, such as drying of the mucus membrane, dry mouth, blurred vision, dizziness, constipation, and urinary hesitancies. In some people, the use of the drug leads to weight gain. It is reasonably well-tolerated by patients and is recommended for depression following a heart attack and stroke. It has a large therapeutic window or effective dosage range and is commonly utilized by psychiatric physicians.

Desipramine has been used to treat people during cocaine withdrawal and those people suffering from attention-deficit disorders, such as an inability to concentrate. Because of its sedating qualities, *only when necessary* should you drive a car or operate machinery or do anything requiring alertness and good motor coordination. If you experience constipation, increase your fluids; and if it persists, ask your doctor about a stool softener or laxative. If you have dry mouth, sugarless hard candy or chewing gum should bring adequate relief.

When preparing to discontinue its use, do not stop abruptly: this can cause withdrawal symptoms, such as irritability, restlessness, nausea, and malaise. These symptoms are annoying, but they are not signs of an addiction.

Pregnancy: Category C (see sidebar on page 69). This means that whatever risk the drug could conceivably pose for the fetus is outweighed by the possible benefits of the drug to the mother. However,

it is advised to avoid its use during the first trimester of a pregnancy, whenever possible.

———————

Brand Name
PAMELOR, AVENTYL

Generic Name
nortriptyline (nor-TRIP-ti-leen)

HOW THE DRUG WORKS

By increasing the amount of norepinephrine or serotonin (or both) in the central nervous system, it improves nerve transmission.

PURPOSE

Depression, especially of a biological origin.

DOSAGE

Treatment of depression
Adults: (initially) 25 mg (taken orally) daily in divided doses, followed by increases, as needed, up to 100 mg daily.
Adolescents and Elderly: 30 mg to 50 mg daily in divided doses.

SIDE EFFECTS

Common: Dizziness; drowsiness; dry mouth; excessive sweating; weight gain; fatigue.
Uncommon: Constipation; diarrhea; vomiting.

ADVERSE REACTIONS

Blurred vision; skin rash; decreased sexual ability; anxiety; restlessness; eye pain; urinary retention; breast enlargement (in males); galactorrhea; trembling; unsteadiness; rapid heart beat; insomnia; nightmares.

DRUG INTERACTION

Increases the effects of drugs such as alcohol and other CNS depressants; narcotic analgesics; amphetaminelike drugs; atropine; oral anticoagulants.
Decreases the effects of clonidine and other antidepressant drugs.

With barbiturates, the effectiveness of the drug decreases.

With MAO inhibitors, fever, delirium, severe excitation, seizures, or death may occur.
With epinephrine or norepinephrine, an increase in blood pressure may occur.

OVERDOSAGE

If any of the following symptoms develops, notify your physician immediately: Drowsiness; cold skin; congestive heart failure; fever; hallucinations; shortness of breath; muscle rigidity; vomiting.

Comments: A derivative of amitriptyline, this drug has slightly more anticholinergic side effects, such as drying of the mucus membrane, dry mouth, blurred vision, dizziness, constipation, and urinary hesitancies. At the same time, it is less sedating than desipramine. It also comes in a lower dose range than desipramine—from 50 to 150 mg—which means less medicine, fewer metabolites, and fewer side effects or adverse reactions.

Although the sedating qualities of nortriptyline are weaker than many other antidepressants, it is important that only when necessary should you drive a car or operate machinery that requires alertness and good motor coordination. When preparing to discontinue its use, do not stop abruptly: it can cause withdrawal symptoms, such as irritability, restlessness, nausea, and malaise. These symptoms are annoying, but they are not signs of an addiction. If you experience constipation, increase your fluids; and if it persists, ask your doctor about a stool softener or laxative. If you have dry mouth, sugarless hard candy or chewing gum should bring adequate relief.

Pregnancy: Category D (see sidebar on page 69). This means that studies in pregnant women have shown a significant risk to the fetus. Therefore, the drug should be used only if needed in a serious disease and when other, safer drugs have proven to be ineffective or cannot be used.

Brand Name	*Generic Name*
VIVACTIL, NEOACTIL	protriptyline (pro-TRIP-ti-leen)

HOW THE DRUG WORKS

By increasing the amount of norepinephrine or serotonin (or both) in the central nervous system, it improves nerve transmission.

PURPOSE

Depression, especially of a biological origin.

DOSAGE

Treatment of depression

Adults: (initially) 25 mg (taken orally) daily in divided doses, followed by increases, as needed, up to 100 mg daily.

Adolescents and Elderly: 30 mg to 50 mg daily in divided doses.

SIDE EFFECTS

Common: Dizziness; drowsiness; dry mouth; excessive sweating; weight gain; fatigue.

Uncommon: Constipation; diarrhea.

ADVERSE REACTIONS

Blurred vision; skin rash; decreased sexual ability; anxiety; restlessness; eye pain; urinary retention; trembling; unsteadiness; rapid heart beat; insomnia.

DRUG INTERACTION

Increases the effects of drugs such as alcohol and other CNS depressants; narcotic analgesics; amphetaminelike drugs; atropine; oral anticoagulants.

Decreases the effects of clonidine and other antidepressant drugs.

With barbiturates, the effectiveness of the drug decreases.

With MAO inhibitors, fevers, delirium, severe excitation, seizures, or death may occur.

With epinephrine or norepinephrine, an increase in blood pressure may occur.

OVERDOSAGE

If any of the following symptoms develops, notify your physician immediately: Drowsiness; cold skin; congestive heart failure; fever; hallucinations; shortness of breath; muscle rigidity; vomiting.

Comments: Protriptyline is the least sedating of drugs in this family of second-generation tricyclic antidepressants; but it also has the greatest tendency to produce cardiac arrhythmias. All cardiac patients and their physicians must be aware of this side effect, especially when the drug is used by the elderly.

Some doctors will prescribe protriptyline to patients whose lethargy causes them to be clinically withdrawn, or for those people who are unable to function normally because of an unexplained lack of energy. Many doctors use it to treat a primary sleep disorder called *obstructive sleep apnea*, a sometimes serious disorder that causes someone to stop breathing for moments during sleep.

Like its sister drug (nortriptyline), protriptyline has high anticholinergic side effects, such as drying of the mucus membrane, dry mouth, blurred vision, dizziness, constipation, and urinary hesitancies. Since it may produce some amphetaminelike effects (stimulant), take it four to six hours before bedtime to avoid insomnia. Nevertheless, it has the lowest dosage range (between 15 mg and 60 mg), which means less medicine, fewer metabolites, and fewer likely side effects or adverse reactions.

If you experience constipation, increase your fluids; if it persists, ask your doctor about a stool softener or laxative. If you have dry mouth, sugarless hard candy or chewing gum should bring adequate relief.

Pregnancy: Category C (see sidebar on page 69). This means that whatever risk the drug could conceivably pose for the fetus is outweighed by the possible benefits of the drug to the mother. However, you are advised to avoid its use during the first trimester of a pregnancy, whenever possible.

Brand Name
SURMONTIL

Generic Name
trimipramine (trye-MIP-ra-meen)

HOW THE DRUG WORKS

By increasing the amount of norepinephrine or serotonin (or both) in the central nervous system, it improves nerve transmission.

PURPOSE

Depression.

DOSAGE

Treatment of depression
 Adults: (initially) 75 mg (taken orally) daily in divided doses, followed by increases, as needed, up to 200 mg daily in divided doses.
 Adolescents and Elderly: (initially) 25 mg to 50 mg daily in single or divided doses, followed by increases, as needed, up to 100 mg daily in divided doses.

SIDE EFFECTS

 Common: Dizziness; drowsiness; dry mouth; excessive sweating; weight gain; fatigue.
 Uncommon: Constipation; diarrhea.

ADVERSE REACTIONS

Blurred vision; skin rash; decreased sexual ability; anxiety; restlessness; eye pain; urinary retention; trembling; unsteadiness; rapid heart beat; insomnia.

DRUG INTERACTION

Increases the effects of drugs such as alcohol and other CNS depressants; narcotic analgesics; amphetaminelike drugs; atropine; oral anticoagulants.
Decreases the effects of clonidine and other antidepressant drugs.

With barbiturates, the effectiveness of the drug decreases.

With MAO inhibitors, fevers, delirium, severe excitation, seizures, or death may occur.

With epinephrine or norepinephrine, an increase in blood pressure may occur.

OVERDOSAGE

If any of the following symptoms develops, notify your physician immediately: Drowsiness; cold skin; congestive heart failure; fever; hallucinations; shortness of breath; muscle rigidity; vomiting.

Comments: Although it has side effects that are similar to desipramine, trimipramine is less commonly used than the other drugs, perhaps because it was the most recently marketed (1987) in this group. Some doctors like to prescribe it with other medications in the treatment of peptic ulcers; but since it has a tendency to produce cardiac arrhythmias, all cardiac patients and their physicians must be aware of this side effect, especially when the drug is used among the elderly.

When preparing to discontinue its use, do not stop abruptly: this can cause withdrawal symptoms, such as irritability, restlessness, nausea, and malaise. These symptoms are annoying but they are not signs of an addiction.

Although it has relatively low sedating qualities, it is important that only when necessary should you drive a car or operate machinery that requires alertness and good motor coordination. If you experience constipation, increase your fluids; and if it persists, ask your doctor about a stool softener or laxative. If you have dry mouth, sugarless hard candy or chewing gum should bring adequate relief.

Pregnancy: Category C (see sidebar on page 69). This means that whatever risk the drug could conceivably pose for the fetus is outweighed by the possible benefits of the drug to the mother. However, you are advised to avoid its use during the first trimester of a pregnancy, whenever possible.

Brand Name	*Generic Name*
ASENDIN	amoxapine (a-MOX-a-peen)

HOW THE DRUG WORKS

By increasing the amount of norepinephrine or serotonin (or both) in the central nervous system, it improves nerve transmission.

PURPOSE

Neurotic depression; depression of a biological origin; psychotic depression; depression associated with anxiety or agitation.

DOSAGE

Treatment of depression
  Adults: (initially) 50 mg (taken orally) daily in divided doses, followed by, if tolerated, up to 100 mg daily in divided doses, by the end of the first week; the usual maintenance dosage is 200 mg to 300 mg daily taken as a single dose at bedtime.
  Elderly: (initially) 25 mg (taken orally) daily, in divided doses, followed, if tolerated, by increments of 50 mg two or three times a day (up to 150 mg daily) by the end of the first week; the usual maintenance dosage is 200 mg to 300 mg daily taken as a single dose at bedtime.

SIDE EFFECTS

  Common: Drowsiness; dry mouth; constipation; blurred vision.
  Uncommon: Diarrhea; anxiety; insomnia; confusion; nervousness; dizziness; increased appetite; increased sweating.

ADVERSE REACTIONS

Tardive dyskinesia (especially in the elderly); skin rash; decreased sexual ability; loss of concentration; restlessness; urinary retention; trembling; seizures; unsteadiness; rapid heartbeat.

DRUG INTERACTION

Increases the effects of drugs such as alcohol and other CNS depressants; narcotic analgesics; amphetaminelike drugs; atropine; oral anticoagulants.
Decreases the effects of clonidine and other antidepressant drugs.

With barbiturates, the effectiveness of the drug decreases.

With MAO inhibitors, fevers, delirium, severe excitation, seizures, or death may occur.

With epinephrine or norepinephrine, an increase in blood pressure may occur.

OVERDOSAGE

If any of the following symptoms develops, notify your physician immediately: Grand mal convulsions; epilepticlike symptoms; coma.

Comments: One of the positive attributes of amoxapine is that it is thought to act more quickly than the other tricyclic antidepressants. In some instances, its effects may occur as soon as four to seven days after its initial use, and almost always within a two-week period.

In addition to most of the symptoms that other tricyclic antidepressants display, the drug can (if used over many months) cause tardive dyskinesia, such as slow, measured, automatic movements, especially in elderly women. Another potential adverse reaction is grand mal seizures, and these symptoms appear to be dose-related: the more you take, the greater the risk. Hence, its use is not recommended for people with a preexisting neurological disease.

Although it has relatively low sedating qualities—except at high doses—it is important that only when necessary should you drive a car or operate machinery that requires alertness and good motor coordination. If you experience constipation, increase your fluids; and if it persists, ask your doctor about a stool softener or laxative. If you have dry mouth, sugarless hard candy or chewing gum should bring adequate relief.

When preparing to discontinue its use, do not stop abruptly: this can cause withdrawal symptoms, such as irritability, restlessness, nausea, and malaise. These symptoms are annoying, but they are not signs of an addiction.

Pregnancy: Category C (see sidebar on page 69). This means that whatever risk the drug could conceivably pose for the fetus is outweighed by the possible benefits of the drug to the mother. However, you are advised to avoid its use during the first trimester of a pregnancy, whenever possible.

Brand Name	*Generic Name*
SINEQUAN, ADAPIN	doxepin (DOX-e-pin)

HOW THE DRUG WORKS

By increasing the amount of norepinephrine or serotonin (or both) in the central nervous system, it improves nerve transmission.

PURPOSE

Psychoneurotic anxiety and/or depression; mixed symptoms of anxiety and depression; anxiety or depression associated with alcoholism; anxiety associated with organic disease; depression accompanied by anxiety or agitation.

DOSAGE

Treatment of depression

Adults: Mild to moderate symptoms: begin with 25 mg (taken orally) daily in divided doses, followed by increases, if necessary; usual maximum dosage is 75 mg to 150 mg daily. Severe symptoms: begin with 50 mg daily in divided doses, followed by gradual increases, up to 300 mg daily, if needed.

Elderly: (initially) 10 mg to 25 mg (taken orally) daily in divided doses, followed, if tolerated, by increments of 50 mg two or three times a day (up to 150 mg daily) by the end of the first week; the usual maintenance dosage is 200 mg to 300 mg daily taken as a single dose at bedtime.

SIDE EFFECTS

Common: Drowsiness; dry mouth; constipation.

Uncommon: Diarrhea; anxiety; insomnia; blurred vision; confusion; nervousness; dizziness; increased appetite; increased sweating; stomach upset; weight gain; hangover.

ADVERSE REACTIONS

Skin rash; edema; decreased sexual ability; loss of concentration; restlessness; urinary retention; trembling; unsteadiness; rapid heartbeat; flushing; chills.

DRUG INTERACTION

Increases the effects of drugs such as alcohol and other CNS depressants; narcotic analgesics; amphetaminelike drugs; atropine; oral anticoagulants.

Decreases the effects of clonidine and other antidepressant drugs.

With barbiturates, the effectiveness of the drug decreases.

With MAO inhibitors, fever, delirium, severe excitation, seizures, or death may occur.

With epinephrine or norepinephrine, an increase in blood pressure may occur.

OVERDOSAGE

If any of the following symptoms develops, notify your physician immediately: Excessive sedation; extrapyramidal symptoms (e.g., spasms of the neck muscles, severe stiffness of the back muscles, rolling back of the eyes, and convulsions).

Comments: Doxepin is sufficiently sedating so that it can be used at night to enhance sleep; at the same time, in doses of 10 mg, it is tolerated well by the elderly. It also significantly reduces gastric acid so that it can be used effectively in people with gastric illnesses of hyperacidity, such as ulcers and gastritis. Some physicians find it as effective as the antiulcer agents TAGAMET and ZANTAC.

At low doses of 25 mg, the drug has adequately controlled the mild depressive or anxiety symptoms accompanying an organic disease like colitis ulcers in some patients. Its drawback is that (like amitriptyline) it has acetylcholinergic side effects, such as low blood pressure. It also causes an early-morning hangover or sluggishness in some individuals, as well as temporary weight gain. Only when necessary should you drive a car or operate machinery that requires alertness and good motor coordination while taking the drug. If you experience constipation, increase your fluids; and if it persists, ask your doctor about a stool softener or laxative. If you have drymouth, sugarless hard candy or chewing gum should bring adequate relief.

When preparing to discontinue its use, do not stop abruptly: this can cause withdrawal symptoms, such as irritability, restlessness, nausea, and malaise. These symptoms are annoying, but they are not signs of an addiction.

Pregnancy: Category C (see sidebar on page 69). This means that whatever risk the drug could conceivably pose for the fetus is outweighed by the possible benefits of the drug to the mother. However, you are advised to avoid its use during the first trimester of a pregnancy, whenever possible.

Brand Name	*Generic Name*
WELLBUTRIN	bupropion HCl (boo-PRO-pi-un)

HOW THE DRUG WORKS

By increasing the amount of norepinephrine in the central nervous system, it improves nerve transmission.

PURPOSE

Depression; stabilizing agent in manic-depressive diseases.

DOSAGE

Treatment of depression
   Adults: (initially) 100 mg (taken orally) daily, in divided doses, followed by increases, if necessary; usual maximum dosage is 225 mg to 450 mg daily.
   Elderly: Doses should be reduced for the elderly.

SIDE EFFECTS

Common: Drowsiness; dry mouth; constipation.
Uncommon: Diarrhea; anxiety; insomnia; blurred vision; confusion; nervousness; dizziness; increased appetite; increased sweating; stomach upset; weight gain; hangover.

ADVERSE REACTIONS

Seizures; skin rash; edema; decreased sexual ability; loss of concentration; restlessness; urinary retention; trembling; unsteadiness; rapid heartbeat; flushing; chills.

DRUG INTERACTION

Increases the effects of drugs such as alcohol and other CNS depressants; narcotic analgesics; amphetaminelike drugs; atropine; oral anticoagulants.

Decreases the effects of clonidine and other antidepressant drugs.

With barbiturates, the effectiveness of the drug decreases.

With MAO inhibitors, fever, delirium, severe excitation, seizures, or death may occur.

With epinephrine or norepinephrine, an increase in blood pressure may occur.

OVERDOSAGE

If any of the following symptoms develops, notify your physician immediately: Excessive sedation; extrapyramidal symptoms; seizures.

Comments: Newly released in the United States (1989), bupropion is different from the conventional second-generation antidepressants. A major concern is the drug's propensity for producing seizures, particularly as the dose increases. Consequently, the size of the dose is limited—and should never be exceeded. This drug may cause a worsening of tics in children with attention deficit disorder and Gilles de la Tourette's syndrome. Bupropion is probably not a *first-line* drug because of a concern over the possibility of dose-related seizures; hence, it may occupy a narrow niche in the antidepressant armamentarium. One of those functions has been as a stabilizing drug in individuals with rapid changes of mood, so-called *rapid cyclers*. Eighty percent of those patients experiencing sexual dysfunction while taking SSRI medications have shown marked improvement when they were switched to WELLBUTRIN.

When preparing to discontinue its use, do not stop abruptly: this can cause withdrawal symptoms, such as irritability, restlessness, nausea, and malaise. These symptoms are annoying, but they are not signs of an addiction. Only when necessary should you drive a car or operate machinery that requires alertness and good motor coordination. If you experience constipation, increase your fluids; and if it persists, ask your doctor about a stool softener or laxative. If you have dry mouth, sugarless hard candy or chewing gum should bring adequate relief.

Pregnancy: Category C (see sidebar on page 69). This means that whatever risk the drug could conceivably pose for the fetus is outweighed by the possible benefits of the drug to the mother. However, you are advised to avoid its use during the first trimester of a pregnancy, whenever possible.

SEROTONIN REUPTAKE BLOCKERS

These drugs represent the newest class of antidepressant drugs and perhaps the *cleanest*. They are referred to as clean drugs because they usually affect only one of the many nervous systems. Because they are more targeted, they have few of the anticholinergic side effects—such as drying of the mucus membrane (including the mouth), blurred vision, dizziness, constipation, and urinary hesitancies—seen in the more conventional first- and second-generation antidepressants.

Serotonin reuptake blockers have the following assets: they have a high degree of effectiveness, tolerable side effects, and one drug, PROZAC, can be taken in a single dose each day. Moreover, they have a wide applicability to a number of conditions other than antidepressants, such as treating substance abuse, obsessive-compulsive disorders (e.g., eating disorders), and panic reactions.

When used with betablockers to treat hypertension, for example, these medications will increase the likelihood of a slowed heartbeat. They will also raise the level of nonsedating antihistamine medications such as SELDANE and HISMANAL and cause heart-rhythm problems. These drugs may also aggravate symptoms of early Parkinson's disease in those people who suffer from the disorder, or cause side effects that give the appearance of the disease. But unlike other classes of drugs, if one SSRI drug is not effective, you can try another drug of that same class. For example, if you were not getting good results from PROZAC, you might have more success with ZOLOFT.

It should be noted that there still are many depressed people who do not respond to these drugs and for whom other medications or strategies may be more appropriate.

Brand Name	Generic Name
DESYREL	trazodone (TRAZ-o-done)

HOW THE DRUG WORKS

By delaying its reuptake, the drug makes the neurotransmitter serotonin more available, thus relieving the symptoms of depression.

PURPOSE

Depression with or without noticeable anxiety.

DOSAGE

Treatment of depression

Adults: (initially) 150 mg (taken orally) daily in divided doses, followed by an increase of, if necessary, 50 mg daily every three to four days, up to 400 mg daily in divided doses, if needed. The maximum dosage is 600 mg for the most severely depressed patient (who is usually hospitalized).

SIDE EFFECTS

Common: Drowsiness; dizziness.

Uncommon: Diarrhea; dry mouth; constipation; anxiety; insomnia; blurred vision; ringing in the ears; confusion; nervousness; increased appetite; weight gain; sweating.

ADVERSE REACTIONS

Skin rash; edema; decreased sexual ability; priapism; nausea; vomiting; restlessness; urinary retention; trembling; unsteadiness; rapid heartbeat.

DRUG INTERACTION

Increases the effects of drugs such as alcohol and other CNS depressants; narcotic analgesics; amphetaminelike drugs; atropine; oral anticoagulants; antihypertensive drugs; digoxin; phenytoin.

OVERDOSAGE

If any of the following symptoms develops, notify your physician immediately: Vomiting; drowsiness; difficulty breathing.

Comments: The first drug in this family, trazodone has a minimal effect on heart function and is safer than the more conventional antidepressants. It also has a sedating quality which makes it effective at night in enhancing sleep. It may also be used in conjunction with PROZAC to counter the insomnia that is frequently associated with the use of that drug. For the same reason, if daytime drowsiness becomes troubling, take the major portion of the drug at bedtime.

It should be taken shortly after a meal or a light snack since more of the drug may be absorbed than when taken on an empty stomach. It may also reduce the likelihood of lightheadedness or dizziness. Because of its sedation, you must exercise considerable caution when driving a car or operating machinery that requires alertness and good motor coordination.

It seems to be of limited efficacy—particularly with the more severe forms of depression. It too has one disconcerting (although relatively rare) side effect: *priapism* (constant erection). If this symptom should occur, see your doctor immediately.

Pregnancy: Category C (see sidebar on page 69). This means that whatever risk the drug could conceivably pose for the fetus is outweighed by the possible benefits of the drug to the mother. However, you are advised to avoid its use during the first trimester of a pregnancy, whenever possible.

Brand Name	Generic Name
PROZAC	fluoxetine (floo-OX-i-teen)

HOW THE DRUG WORKS

By delaying its reuptake, the drug makes the neurotransmitter serotonin more available, thus relieving the symptoms of depression.

PURPOSE

Depression.

DOSAGE

Treatment of depression
Adults: (initially) 20 mg (taken orally) each morning; after several weeks, if needed, increase to 80 mg daily in divided doses (morning and evening).

SIDE EFFECTS

Common: Headaches; nervousness; anxiety; nausea; insomnia; drowsiness; dizziness; diarrhea; dry mouth; dyspepsia; excessive sweating.

Uncommon: Constipation; abdominal pain; flatulence; vomiting; weight loss; tremor; taste change; hot flashes; flulike symptoms; sinusitis; sore throat; nasal congestion; fatigue; sedation; abnormal dreams; decreased concentration; alopecia (hair loss).

ADVERSE REACTIONS

Skin rash; chest pain; ear pain; painful menstruation; sexual dysfunction; back pain; palpitation; angina pectoris; akathisia; impaired urination; abnormal gait; incontinence.

DRUG INTERACTION

Increases the half-life of diazepam.

With warfarin and digitoxin (drugs that are tightly bound to plasma proteins), it can cause toxic effects.

With tryptophan, it will cause restlessness, agitation, and GI distress.

With DILATIN, it will raise the DILATIN blood level. Use only with low levels of LITHIUM because it will raise blood level of LITHIUM.

With alprazolam (XANAX), it will prolong its half-life by 50 percent (more will remain). Thus, to treat anxiety, clonazepam is a better choice as PROZAC has no effect on that drug.

OVERDOSAGE

If any of the following symptoms develops, notify your physician immediately: Vomiting; nausea; agitation; restlessness (and other signs of excited CNS); seizures.

Comments: PROZAC is arguably the ideal drug, to date. It has 80 percent efficacy, and the vast majority of patients respond to a single dose, usually one pill in the morning (at least to begin with). Its other favorable features are: it is nonsedating, does not cause weight gain, has few cardiovascular effects, and has a wide range of efficacy. Recent studies have also suggested that it may alter the craving for alcohol and other addicting drugs. It also has been utilized in eating disorders, particularly bulimia. And at a higher dosage range of 40 mg to 80 mg, it has been found to be effective in suppressing symptoms of obsessive-compulsive disorders.

PROZAC has also now been approved for the treatment of obsessive-compulsive disorders, as have the drugs ANAFRANIL and LUVOX.

Some individuals used PROZAC informally as a weight-loss drug. This is ill-advised, if for no other reason than studies indicate that while one-third of all users will lose weight, another third will increase theirs, and, for the balance, the drug will not have an effect at all.

Most of the disconcerting side effects are relatively short-lasting. The insomnia it causes can be treated with the addition of either trazodone or a short-acting benzodiazepine hypnotic at night for the first few days to counter the symptom. If possible, you are also advised to avoid taking the drug in the afternoon to prevent sleep disturbances. Individuals with coexisting anxiety and depression may find the restlessness or nervousness difficult to tolerate. Augmentation with a short-acting benzodiazepine, such as alprazolam, may be effective in averting this disconcerting side effect.

The antidepressant effects may take four weeks or longer to fully develop. At the same time, it has a long half-life (which means it can be given every other day); it remains in the body up to 50 hours after its ingestion. Consequently, a washout period of as long as one week has been recommended when changing from this drug to conventional tricyclic antidepressants. A longer washout period may be necessary when shifting from monoamine-oxidase (MAO) inhibitor antidepressants to PROZAC.

Pregnancy: Category B (see sidebar on page 69). This means that the risk to the fetus is relatively low. PROZAC is not recommended for nursing mothers as it can cause irritability in the infant and increase its heart and respiration rate.

Brand Name
ANAFRANIL

Generic Name
clomipramine (klo-MIP-ra-meen)

HOW THE DRUG WORKS

By delaying its reuptake, the drug makes the neurotransmitter serotonin more available, thus relieving the symptoms of depression.

PURPOSE

Depression associated with anxiety and obsessive-compulsive neurosis.

DOSAGE

Treatment of depression

Adults: (initially) 25 mg (taken orally) daily in divided doses, increasing to a maximum of 150 mg daily; severely depressed patients may take up to 300 mg daily.

Elderly and Debilitated Patients: (initially) 20 mg to 30 mg daily in divided doses, with gradual increases as needed.

SIDE EFFECTS

Common: Headaches; nervousness; nausea; drowsiness; dizziness; dry mouth; tiredness; weight gain.

Uncommon: Diarrhea; excessive sweating; heartburn; blurred vision; vomiting.

ADVERSE REACTIONS

Skin rash; chest pain; ear pain; irregular menstruation and sexual dysfunction; breast enlargement and galactorrhea in females; gynecomastia in males; jaundice; urine retention; disorientation; extrapyramidal reactions; convulsions.

DRUG INTERACTION

Increases the effects of drugs such as alcohol and other CNS depressants.

Decreases the effectiveness of antihypertensives.

With MAO inhibitors, it may cause adverse reactions.

With thyroid medications, it may increase the risk of dysrhythmia.

With ACE inhibitors (antihypertensive drugs), will increase levels of ANAFRANIL and its side effects.

OVERDOSAGE

If any of the following symptoms develops, notify your physician immediately: Vomiting; nausea; agitation; restlessness (and other signs of excited CNS); seizures.

Comments: Although introduced in Switzerland in 1966, France in 1967, and England in 1970, ANAFRANIL has only been allowed to be sold here in 1990. The delay in marketing the drug in this country centered on its potential risk of causing grand mal seizures. Despite this potential risk, it remains one of the most effective drugs in the treatment of obsessive-compulsive diseases. It is especially recommended for people who are suffering from an obsessive-compulsive disorder or depression.

A washout period of as long as two weeks is recommended when shifting from monoamine-oxidase (MAO) inhibitor antidepressants to this drug. You may experience urine retention and, if constipation becomes a problem, a stool softener should provide some relief. The nuisance of dry mouth may be helped by sugarless hard candy or chewing gum. The drug has a mild sedating effect; therefore it is advised that if you must drive a car or operate machinery that requires alertness or good coordination, you do so with considerable caution.

Pregnancy: Category not yet established.

Brand Name	Generic Name
LUVOX	fluvoxamine (floo-VOX-a-meen)

HOW THE DRUG WORKS

By selectively blocking the reuptake of the neurotransmitter serotonin.

PURPOSE

Diminish and eliminate repetitive and intrusive thoughts and behaviors.

DOSAGE

Adults: (Initially) 50 mg with increments of 50 mg to maximum levels of 100 mg to 300 mg.

SIDE EFFECTS

Common: Nausea; sleepiness; insomnia; nervousness; dry mouth.
Uncommon: Constipation; weight loss; sore throat; nasal congestion; fatigue; sedation; abdominal pain; vomiting; tremor; flulike symptoms; flatulence.

ADVERSE REACTIONS

Seizures have been reported during LUVOX administration.

DRUG INTERACTION

When taken with antihistamines, terfenadine (SELDANE) and astemizole (HISMANAL), it slows the heart rate.

Drug should not be used with monoamine oxidase antidepressants or those in the tricyclic family.

Should be used with caution if used with warfarin, phenytoin (antiseizure medication), and the cardiac arrythymics of the betablocker family, CORGARD and VISKEN, because it may elevate the blood levels, causing overdoses.

OVERDOSAGE

If any of the following symptoms develop, notify your physician immediately: Somnolence; dizziness; gastrointestinal complaints, such as nausea, vomiting, and diarrhea.

Comments: Currently, LUVOX is approved solely for its anti-obsessive effect. Like its sister drugs, fluoxetine and clomipramine, it also effectively treats both antidepressant and obsessive symptoms and was originally marketed as an antidepressant. However, unlike fluoxetine, it is short acting since it has no active metabolites and is less likely to cause insomnia. The medication also has no anticholinergic side effects such as dry mouth or blurry vision.

LUVOX should be used with caution if you have any pre-existing seizure disorders. The medication also should not be used with alcohol because it may lead to increased levels of psychomotor impairment.

Pregnancy: Category B (see sidebar on page 69). This means that the risk to the fetus is assumed to be relatively low. The effects of this drug during pregnancy, however, have not been studied. Hence, notify your doctor if you plan to become pregnant.

Brand Name	Generic Name
LUDIOMIL	maprotiline (ma-PRO-ti-leen)

HOW THE DRUG WORKS

By delaying its reuptake, the drug makes the neurotransmitter serotonin more available, thus relieving the symptoms of depression.

PURPOSE

Depressive illness with depressive anxiety and manic-depressive illness; anxiety associated with depression.

DOSAGE

Treatment of depression

Adults: (initially) 75 mg (taken orally) daily in a single dose or divided doses for two weeks *in patients with mild to moderate depression*; doses can be gradually increased, if needed, in 25-mg increments to a maximum dosage of 150 mg daily; *in the most severely depressed hospitalized patients*, 100 mg to 150 mg daily in a single dose or divided doses up to a maximum of 225 mg.

Elderly and Debilitated Patients: (initially) 25 mg daily, followed by gradual increases, if needed.

SIDE EFFECTS

Common: Dry mouth; drowsiness, dizziness; nervousness; headaches; tiredness; blurred vision; insomnia.

Uncommon: Constipation; diarrhea; heartburn; sensitivity to the sun; excessive sweating.

ADVERSE REACTIONS

Severe constipation; vomiting; seizures; itchy skin rash; trembling; weight loss; excitability. *Rare:* Confusion; hallucinations; irregular heartbeat; sore throat and fever; yellowing of the eyes (jaundice).

DRUG INTERACTION

Barbiturates, methylphenidate, and cemetidine increase the effects of the drug.

With MAO inhibitors, it may cause adverse reactions (including seizures).

OVERDOSAGE

If any of the following symptoms develops, notify your physician immediately: Profound dizziness and sleepiness; fever; severe muscle stiffness; rapid heartbeat.

Comments: LUDIOMIL can cause an increased sensitivity to the skin. Hence, avoid prolonged exposure to the sun, especially during the hours of 11 A.M. to 2 P.M.; when in the sun, use a sunscreen and wear protective clothing. A washout period of as long as two weeks is recommended when changing from monoamine-oxidase (MAO) inhibitors to this drug.

The drug has a mild sedating effect. Therefore it is advised that, if you must drive a car or operate machinery that requires alertness or good coordination, you do so with considerable caution. The nuisance of dry mouth may be helped by sugarless hard candy or chewing gum.

Pregnancy: Category B (see sidebar on page 69). This means that the risk to the fetus is relatively low.

Brand Name	*Generic Name*
EFFEXOR	venlafaxine (ven-la-FAX-een)

HOW THE DRUG WORKS

By preventing the reuptake of both serotonin and norepinephrine neurotransmitters. It is also a weak inhibitor of dopamine reuptake.

PURPOSE

Depression.

DOSAGE

Treatment of depression

Adults: (initially) 75 mg per day (taken orally), given as 25-mg doses three times a day. The maximum dose is 375 mg per day in an inpatient setting.

Adolescents and Elderly: The effectiveness and safety for children and the elderly has not been established.

SIDE EFFECTS

Common: Dry mouth; weakness; sweating; nausea; diarrhea, dizziness; constipation; abnormal dreams.

Uncommon: Light-headedness; loss of appetite; decreased sexual drive.

ADVERSE REACTIONS

High blood pressure; agitation; sleepiness; feelings of worthlessness. *Rare:* seizures.

DRUG INTERACTION

Increases the effects of LITHIUM, VALIUM, and other tranquilizers, narcotic painkillers, and alcohol. This drug should not be taken with MAO inhibitor drugs.

Consult your physician before combining with other antidepressants, or OTC sleep aids.

OVERDOSAGE

If any of the following symptoms develop, notify your physician immediately: Somnolence (excessive sleepiness); seizures; abnormal heart rhythm.

Comments: Introduced in 1993, the appeal of EFFEXOR is that it acts more rapidly in the treatment of depression, usually within two weeks of scheduled use, but with fewer of the sedative and cardiovascular side effects associated with other antidepressants currently available. Long-term use of the drug may require your doctor to adjust your dosage at various times.

You should notify your doctor before taking this drug if you suffer from hypertension (high blood pressure), heart, kidney, or liver disease, or have had a history of seizures or manic behaviors. People with diminished kidney function may have their dosage reduced and those with diminished liver function may be able to tolerate only half or less of the usual dosage. If you experience hives while taking this drug, notify your doctor.

When preparing to discontinue its use, do not stop abruptly. This can result in withdrawal symptoms, such as restlessness, irritability, and insomnia. A washout period of fourteen days is also recommended when shifting from an MAO inhibitor to EFFEXOR.

You should drive a car or operate machinery that requires alertness and good motor coordination only when necessary while taking this drug. If you have dry mouth, sugarless hard candy or chewing gum should bring adequate relief.

Pregnancy: Category C (see sidebar on page 69). This means that whatever risk the drug could conceivably pose for the fetus is outweighed by the possible benefits of the drug to the mother. However, if you plan to become pregnant, notify your doctor as it is advised to avoid its use during the first trimester of a pregnancy when possible.

Brand Name	*Generic Name*
ZOLOFT	sertraline (SER-tra-leen)

HOW THE DRUG WORKS

By inhibiting the reuptake of the neurotransmitter serotonin. Because it has little or no effect on other neurotransmitters, it is considered an SSRI (selective serotonin reuptake inhibitor).

PURPOSE

Symptomatic relief of depressive illness.

DOSAGE

Treatment of depression

Adults: (initially) 50 mg (taken orally) daily, in the morning, and increase gradually, 50 mg intervals each week if needed. The maximum dosage should not exceed 200 mg per day.

Adolescents and Elderly: The effectiveness and safety for children and the elderly has not been established.

SIDE EFFECTS

Common: Headache; insomnia; drowsiness; fatigue; dizziness; nervousness; constipation; weakness; abdominal pain; nausea; diarrhea, and dyspepsia.

Uncommon: Dry mouth; wheezing; rash; anaphylaxis (severe allergic reaction); sexual dysfunction (in the form of ejaculatory delay).

ADVERSE REACTIONS

Confusion; irritability; chills; fever; allergic reactions; and muscle rigidity. *Rare:* dermatitis.

DRUG INTERACTION

Increases the effects of diazepam, warfarin, and tolbutamide (an oral antidiabetic medication).

If taken with insulin or hypoglycemic medications, it may increase risk of hypoglycemic reaction.

If taken with cimetidine (antacid inhibitor), it will increase blood levels of sertraline.

OVERDOSAGE

If any of the following symptoms develop, notify your physician immediately: Somnolence; nausea; vomiting; rapid heartbeat; agitation; restlessness; and seizures.

Comments: Sertraline was not accepted by the FDA until 1993–94 and is now a commonly used alternative to PROZAC (fluoxetine).

The drug's side effect, sedation, helps patients suffering from severe insomnia. Lacking the notoriety of PROZAC and its sometimes jarring side effects, sertraline appears to be more acceptable to patients, though some people report a slight weight loss with use of it. Caution must be exercised in patients with bipolar mood disorders to avoid triggering a manic episode (a shift of mood and energy level). Since adverse reactions have been reported in those patients who began MAO inhibitor antidepressants without an intervening waiting period, a washout or waiting period of two to five weeks is recommended when shifting from MAO inhibitors to this drug.

Pregnancy: Category B (see sidebar on page 69). This means that the risk to the fetus is relatively low.

Brand Name	*Generic Name*
PAXIL	paroxetine (pair-o-SET-een)

HOW THE DRUG WORKS

By selectively inhibiting the reuptake of serotonin, it reduces the symptoms of depression.

PURPOSE

Symptomatic relief of mild to moderately severe depression.

DOSAGE

Treatment of depression
Adults: (initially) 20 mg (taken orally) daily, usually in the morning. Although this dose is generally effective, increments of 10 mg can be added until a total dose of 50 mg per day is reached.
Elderly (or those with kidney and liver disease): Begin with 10 mg; maximum dosage should not exceed 40 mg.

SIDE EFFECTS

Common: Dry mouth; nausea; sleepiness; sweating; and sexual dysfunction (in the form of ejaculatory delay).

Uncommon: Headaches; dizziness; increased appetite; allergic reactions.

ADVERSE REACTIONS

Hyperventilation; protracted nausea; and weakness.

DRUG INTERACTION

Increases effects of warfarin and other antidepressants, major tranquillizers, anticonvulsants, and antiarrythmics.

If taken with cimetidine (antacid inhibitor), will increase blood level of paroxetine.

OVERDOSAGE

If any of the following symptoms develop, notify your physician immediately: Slow heartbeat; vomiting; tremor; feeling of persecution; convulsions.

Comments: The symptoms of depression should lessen within a month of using paroxetine. Because this drug tends to be sedating, it is frequently used in patients with prominent agitation and could be used in single-night doses for patients with insomnia. The drug should be used with great caution in patients with a history of cardiovascular disease, seizures, and manic disorders. Notify your doctor, also, if you have a history of liver or kidney disease.

When preparing to discontinue its use, do not stop abruptly. This can result in withdrawal symptoms, such as restlessness, irritability, and insomnia. A washout period of fourteen days is also recommended when shifting from MAO inhibitors to PAXIL. You should drive a car or operate machinery that requires alertness and good motor coordination only when necessary while taking this drug. Do not drink alcohol while taking this drug or take antacids two hours before or after taking this drug. Dry mouth can be relieved with sugarless gum or hard candy.

Pregnancy: Category B (see sidebar on page 69). This means that the risk to the fetus is assumed to be relatively low. The effects of this drug during pregnancy, however, have not been studied. Hence, notify your doctor if you plan to become pregnant. Because the drug appears in breast milk and might affect a nursing infant, it is recommended that mothers do not breast-feed while using the drug.

Brand Name	*Generic Name*
SERZONE	nefazadone (ne-FAZ-a-doan)

HOW THE DRUG WORKS

By promoting the transmission of serotonin, using two separate pathways, the drug both selectively blocks some serotonin receptors and inhibits the reuptake of serotonin in others. SERZONE also inhibits the reuptake of norepinephrine, a new and novel characteristic of the drug.

PURPOSE

Treatment of depression.

DOSAGE

Treatment of depression
   Adults: (Initially) 200 mg daily, given in two doses. Increments of 100 mg to 200 mg per day can be added until an effective dose can be established. Therapeutic doses are usually between 300 mg and 600 mg per day.

SIDE EFFECTS

Common: Dry mouth; nausea; sleepiness.
Uncommon: Abdominal pain; syncope; gastrointestinal bleeding.

ADVERSE REACTIONS

Laboratory studies have indicated an increased level of the hormone prolactin. In male patients this means painful breasts with discharge or lactorrhea. Similar studies have not been done in females, but they are probably at risk for lactorrhea, abnormal menses, and weight gain. Increased prolactin may also be detrimental in women with present or past histories of breast cancer.

DRUG INTERACTION

Concomitant use of nefazodone with alprazolam or triazolam may lead to psychomotor impairment because their unique metabolism may lead to increased blood levels of the drugs. Other drugs with similar metabolic pathways include the cardiac drugs nifedipine, quinidine, lidocaine, and erythromycin and should be used with caution.

Nefazadone should not be used with the antihistamine terfenadine (SELDANE) or astemizole (HISMANAL) because it blocks the metabolism of these two drugs and seriously slows the heart rate.

OVERDOSAGE

If any of the following symptoms develop, notify your physician immediately: Excessive sedation; weakness; confusion; agitation.

Comments: Initial experience indicates that nefazadone produces no sexual difficulties like those attributable to SSRI antidepressants, such as the cases of priapism that have been reported with the use of its sister compound, trazodone. The newness of the drug prevents extensive commentary. However, it is thought that the drug may fill a niche by serving those individuals who failed to respond to the previous generation of antidepressants. But there is no comparative data available at this time.

Pregnancy: Category C (see sidebar on page 69). This means that whatever risk the drug could conceivably pose for the fetus is outweighed by the possible benefits of the drug to the mother. However, if you plan to become pregnant, notify your doctor.

MONOAMINE-OXIDASE INHIBITORS

This class of medication was developed quite accidentally from drugs used to treat tuberculosis. The prototype drug, iproniazid, was discontinued because of serious adverse effects on the liver. However, the family that is currently used, the hydralazine family, has less impact on the liver. These drugs interfere with the metabolism of the major chemical messengers in the brain and are very powerful. Even though each drug has a somewhat different profile of side effects, they all require a considerable amount of awareness.

As with many other families of antidepressants, monoamine-oxidase (MAO) inhibitors are used to treat a wide spectrum of disorders, such as panic reactions and various eating disorders. They have a relatively lower dosage range than most other anti-depressant drugs—many as low as 30 to 60 mg per day.

One of the most important adverse effects of these drugs is related to diet. Tyramine, a substance found in some foods, normally undergoes conversion in the body to an inactive form through the action of the enzyme *monoamine-oxidase*. The monoamine-oxidase (MAO) inhibitors treat depression by blocking this enzyme. Consequently, when the MAO drugs are taken, the tyramine remains active and causes the release of the chemical norepinephrine, which, in turn, makes the blood vessels constrict and blood pressure rise. The inadvertent use of the wrong food with these medications can produce symptoms such as severe headaches, nausea, vomiting, and heart palpitations. A stroke or even death can be caused by this food-and-drug interaction.

Hence, the chemical reaction between certain foods and MAO inhibitors requires considerable alertness. For some individuals this will mean going on a diet that is free of a number of favorite foods, such as hot dogs, cheeses, and alcoholic beverages (especially beer, sherry, and Chianti wines).

Another major concern is that many medications, particularly those found in over-the-counter drugs—such as cold medicine, hay fever medication, cough medicine with dextromethorphan—cannot be used in conjunction with these drugs because they act as stimulants. The drug interaction can trigger episodes of extreme exhilaration or paranoia, excitement or manic episodes, or, in individuals with latent psychotic episodes, delusions or hallucinations.

. A third major consideration concerns analgesics or painkillers, particularly meperidine. The combination of these medications may lead to symptoms such as high blood pressure, headache, nausea, and dizziness. In some instances, it can create a major medical emergency.

Because of the restrictions on diet and a wide variety of possible interactions with other sources of hidden pressor agents (i.e., chemicals in nonprescription medications), MAO inhibitors are usually kept as a second-line drug. They are used in situations where someone is not responding to or is generally failing to get relief from other tricyclic medications. They are also used in those instances of so-called *atypical depression*: those depressive symptoms that include overeating and oversleeping. (See "Depression," page 54.) As a family, these drugs are more likely to affect sexual function, particularly sexual arousal and orgasm.

So as not to cause an adverse interaction, these drugs require a washout period of at least two weeks or more following their use before another family of antidepressants can be used.

Brand Name	*Generic Name*
NARDIL	phenelzin (FEN-el-zeen)

HOW THE DRUG WORKS

By inhibiting the action of the enzyme (monoamine-oxidase), this drug produces an increase of the neurotransmitters that preserve normal mood and emotional stability.

PURPOSE

Long-term chronic depression.

DOSAGE

Treatment of depression

Adults: (initially) 15 mg (taken orally) followed by rapid increase—60 mg to 90 mg daily in divided doses; once maximum benefit is reached, reduce dosage slowly over several weeks to 15 mg daily or 15 mg every other day.

SIDE EFFECTS

Common: Drowsiness; dizziness; orthostatic hypotension; weakness; dry mouth; insomnia; trembling; restlessness; increased appetite or weight gain; headache; decreased sexual ability.
Uncommon: Chills; urinary retention; jitters.

ADVERSE REACTIONS

Severe dizziness or light-headedness; diarrhea; edema; pounding heartbeat. *Rare:* dark urine, skin rash, or yellowing of the eyes (suggests drug-induced hepatitis).

Signs of hypertension: Nose bleed; chest pains; enlarged pupils; severe headache; sensitivity to light; nausea and vomiting; feverish sweating.

DRUG INTERACTION

Increases the effects of alcohol, barbiturates, and other CNS sedatives; narcotics; tricyclic antidepressants; dextromethorphan (OTC cough medicines).
Increases risk of high blood pressure with amphetamines, ephedrine, levodopa, meperidine, metaraminol, methotrimeprazine, methylphenidate, phenylephrine, phenylpropanolamine.

OVERDOSAGE

If any of the following symptoms develops, notify your physician immediately: Anxiety; irritability; confusion; clammy, cool skin; fever; hallucinations; agitation; rapid or irregular heartbeat; coma.

Comments: You may not feel the full benefits of NARDIL (the most commonly used MAO) until as much as 60 mg has been taken for a month or more. It should not be used in patients with a history of heart disease, hypertension, kidney or liver disease, or those over the age of sixty. Some doctors prescribe it in the treatment of bulimia.
While taking this drug, avoid tyramine-containing foods (see "Tyramine-Rich Foods," page 88), and do not drink alcohol or self-medicate with cold, hay fever, or weight-reducing preparations. Do not discontinue the drug without your doctor's advice, and maintain

all the food-and-drug restrictions for at least ten days following termination of its use.

The incidence of orthostatic hypotension is high, and you may become dizzy when standing from a sitting or lying position.

Pregnancy: Category C (see sidebar on page 69). This means that whatever risk the drug could conceivably pose for the fetus is outweighed by the possible benefits of the drug to the mother. However, you are advised to avoid its use during the first trimester of a pregnancy, whenever possible.

Brand Name	*Generic Name*
MARPLAN	isocarboxazid (eye-so-kar-BOX-a-zid)

HOW THE DRUG WORKS

By inhibiting the action of the enzyme (monoamine-oxidase), the drug produces an increase of the neurotransmitters that preserve normal mood and emotional stability.

PURPOSE

Long-term chronic depression.

DOSAGE

Treatment of depression

Adults: (initially) 30 mg (taken orally) taken daily in a single dose or in divided doses, followed by a reduction to 10 mg to 20 mg daily (or possibly less) when the condition improves.

Children: This drug is not recommended for children under twelve.

SIDE EFFECTS

Common: Drowsiness; dizziness; orthostatic hypotension; weakness; dry mouth; insomnia; trembling; restlessness; increased appetite or weight gain; headache; decreased sexual ability.

Uncommon: Chills; urinary retention; jitters.

138

ADVERSE REACTIONS

Severe dizziness or light-headedness; diarrhea; edema; pounding heartbeat. *Rare:* dark urine, skin rash, or yellowing of the eyes (suggests drug-induced hepatitis).

Signs of hypertension: Nosebleed; chest pains; enlarged pupils; severe headache; sensitivity to light; nausea and vomiting; feverish sweating.

DRUG INTERACTION

Increases the effects of alcohol, barbiturates, and other CNS sedatives; narcotics; tricyclic antidepressants; dextromethorphan (OTC cough medicines).

Increases risk of high blood pressure with amphetamines, ephedrine, levodopa, meperidine, metaraminol, methotrimeprazine, methylphenidate, phenylephrine, phenylpropanolamine.

OVERDOSAGE

If any of the following symptoms develops, notify your physician immediately: Anxiety; irritability; confusion; clammy, cool skin; fever; hallucinations; agitation; rapid or irregular heartbeat; coma.

Comments: You may not feel the full benefit of MARPLAN for at least two to four weeks. It should not be used in patients with a history of heart disease, hypertension, kidney or liver disease, or those over the age of sixty. Some doctors prescribe it in the treatment of bulimia.

While taking this drug, avoid tyramine-containing foods (see "Tyramine-Rich Foods," page 88), and do not drink alcohol or self-medicate with cold, hay fever, or weight-reducing preparations. Do not discontinue it without your doctor's advice, and maintain all the food-and-drug restrictions for at least ten days following termination of its use.

MARPLAN is thought to have a milder side-effect profile than either phenelzin or tranylcypromine. Nevertheless, its incidence of orthostatic hypotension is still significant, and you may become dizzy when standing from a sitting or lying position.

Pregnancy: Category C (see sidebar on page 69). This means that whatever risk the drug could conceivably pose for the fetus is outweighed by the possible benefits of the drug to the mother. However, you are advised to avoid its use during the first trimester of a pregnancy, whenever possible.

Brand Name PARNATE	*Generic Name* tranylcypromine (tran- ill-SIP-ro-meen)

HOW THE DRUG WORKS

By inhibiting the action of the enzyme (monoamine-oxidase), the drug produces an increase of the neurotransmitters that preserve normal mood and emotional stability.

PURPOSE

Long-term chronic depression, or major depressive episodes.

DOSAGE

Treatment of depression
Adults: (initially) 30 mg (taken orally) daily in divided doses, for two weeks; if no improvement, increase dosage in increments of 10 mg daily at intervals of one to three weeks up to a maximum of 60 mg daily.
Children: This drug is not recommended for children under twelve.

SIDE EFFECTS

Common: Drowsiness; dizziness; orthostatic hypotension; weakness; dry mouth; insomnia; trembling; restlessness; increased appetite or weight gain; headache; decreased sexual ability.
Uncommon: Chills; urinary retention; jitters.

ADVERSE REACTIONS

Severe dizziness or light-headedness; diarrhea; edema; pounding heartbeat. *Rare:* dark urine, skin rash, or yellowing of the eyes (suggests drug-induced hepatitis).

ont2e +

Signs of hypertension: chest pains; enlarged pupils; severe headache; sensitivity to light; nausea and vomiting; feverish sweating.

DRUG INTERACTION

Increases the effects of alcohol, barbiturates, and other CNS sedatives; narcotics; tricyclic antidepressants; dextromethorphan (OTC cough medicines).

Increases risk of high blood pressure with amphetamines, ephedrine, levodopa, meperidine, metaraminol, methotrimeprazine, methylphenidate, phenylephrine, phenylpropanolamine.

OVERDOSAGE

If any of the following symptoms develops, notify your physician immediately: Anxiety; irritability; confusion; clammy, cool skin; fever; hallucinations; agitation; rapid or irregular heartbeat; coma.

Comments: You may not feel the full benefit of PARNATE for at least two to four weeks. This drug should not be used in patients with a history of heart disease, hypertension, kidney or liver disease, or those over the age of sixty. Some doctors prescribe it in the treatment of bulimia.

While taking this drug, avoid tyramine-containing foods (see "Tyramine-Rich Foods," page 88), and do not drink alcohol or self-medicate with cold, hay fever, or weight-reducing preparations. Do not discontinue the drug without your doctor's advice, and maintain all the food-and-drug restrictions for at least ten days following termination of its use.

Following excessive doses, some patients have experienced withdrawal symptoms, such as restlessness, anxiety, depression, confusion, hallucinations, headaches, and diarrhea. Consequently, do not abruptly stop taking the drug, but taper its discontinuance. Also, be aware that the drug can cause a throbbing headache and significant orthostatic hypotension, that is, dizziness when standing from a sitting or lying position.

Pregnancy: Category C (see sidebar on page 69). This means that whatever risk the drug could conceivably pose for the fetus is outweighed by the possible benefits of the drug to the mother. However, you are advised to avoid its use during the first trimester of a pregnancy, whenever possible.

Brand Name	*Generic Name*
EUTONYL	pargyline (PAR-gi-leen)

HOW THE DRUG WORKS

By inhibiting the action of the enzyme (monoamine-oxidase), this drug produces an increase of the neurotransmitters that preserve normal mood and emotional stability.

PURPOSE

Depression.

DOSAGE

Treatment of depression

Adults: (initially) 25 mg (taken orally) daily in single dose; followed by weekly increases of up to 10 mg until desired results are reached, not to exceed 200 mg daily. (In combination with other drugs, maximum dosage is 25 mg.)

Elderly: (initially) 10 mg to 25 mg and the usual daily dosage of 25 mg to 50 mg.

SIDE EFFECTS

Common: Drowsiness; dizziness; orthostatic hypotension; weakness; dry mouth; constipation.

Uncommon: Chills; insomnia; restlessness; shakiness; nightmares; sensitivity to sunlight; increased appetite and weight gain.

ADVERSE REACTIONS

Diarrhea; edema; pounding heartbeat; chest pain; nausea and vomiting; stiff or sore neck. *Rare:* dark urine and yellowing of the eyes (suggests drug-induced hepatitis); fever; hallucinations.

DRUG INTERACTION

Increases the effects of alcohol, barbiturates, and other CNS sedatives; narcotics; tricyclic antidepressants; dextromethorphan (OTC cough medicines).

Increases risk of high blood pressure with amphetamines, ephedrine, levodopa, meperidine, metaraminol, methotrimeprazine, methylphenidate, phenylephrine, phenylpropanolamine.

OVERDOSAGE

If any of the following symptoms develops, notify your physician immediately: Anxiety; irritability; confusion; clammy, cool skin; fever; hallucinations; agitation; rapid or irregular heartbeat; coma.

Comments: Generally used to control hypertension, EUTONYL has also been used successfully to treat depression, especially in those people who have not received symptom relief from other MAO inhibitors. The elderly may be more sensitive to its sedating and hypotensive effects.

You may not feel the full benefits of this drug for the first one or two weeks. It is advised that you take it in the morning to avoid the possibility of insomnia; but no nonprescription cold medicines should be taken with it without your doctor's permission.

You must strictly observe a two-week washout before using another antidepressant medication, such as a tricyclic antidepressant or SSRIs. The danger is that any traces of this drug in your system may interact with the new antidepressant to cause tremors, agitation, seizures, rigidity, and fevers.

Avoid tyramine-containing foods (see page 88), do not drink alcohol or self-medicate with cold, hay fever, or weight-reducing preparations while taking this drug. Do not discontinue it without your doctor's advice, and maintain all the food-and-drug restrictions for at least ten days following termination of its use.

Pregnancy: Category C (see sidebar on page 69). This means that whatever risk the drug could conceivably pose for the fetus is outweighed by the possible benefits of the drug to the mother. However,

you are advised to avoid its use during the first trimester of a pregnancy, whenever possible.

Brand Name
ELDEPRYL

Generic Name
selegiline (sell-e-GILL-een)

HOW THE DRUG WORKS

By suppressing the enzyme monoamine-oxidase (MAO) inhibitor in the brain, this drug increases the activity of dopamine in the CNS.

PURPOSE OF DRUG

Parkinson's disease; augmentation of traditional treatment.

DOSAGE

Treatment of Parkinson's disease
   Adults: 10 mg (taken orally) as a single morning dose or 5 mg in divided doses.

SIDE EFFECTS

   Common: Dizziness; orthostatic hypotension.
   Uncommon: Insomnia; anxiety; nausea; vomiting.

ADVERSE REACTIONS

Dyskinesia (e.g., chewing movements); hallucinations; confusion; agitation.

DRUG INTERACTION

Increases the effects of alcohol, barbiturates, and other CNS sedatives; narcotics; tricyclic antidepressants; dextromethorphan (over-the-counter cough medicines).

Increases risk of high blood pressure with amphetamines, ephedrine, levodopa, meperidine, metaraminol, methotrimeprazine, methylphenidate, phenylephrine, phenylpropanolamine.

OVERDOSAGE

If any of the following symptoms develops, notify your physician immediately: Anxiety; irritability; confusion; clammy, cool skin; fever; hallucinations; agitation; rapid or irregular heartbeat; coma.

Comments: This MAO inhibitor with antidepressant qualities is used in the augmentation of traditional treatment of depression. The elderly may be more sensitive to ELDEPRYL's sedating and hypotensive effects.

You may not feel the full benefits of this drug for the first one or two weeks. You are advised to take it in the morning to avoid the possibility of insomnia.

While it is routinely advised to avoid foods containing tyramine, such as aged cheese (see page 88), while using this drug, patients taking less than 10 mg will not be adversely affected by tyramine-containing foods. Do not drink alcohol or self-medicate with cold, hay fever, or weight-reducing preparations while taking this drug. Do not discontinue it without your doctor's advice, and maintain all the food-and-drug restrictions for at least ten days following termination of its use.

Pregnancy: Category C (see sidebar on page 69). This means that whatever risk the drug could conceivably pose for the fetus is outweighed by the possible benefits of the drug to the mother. However, you are advised to avoid its use during the first trimester of a pregnancy, whenever possible.

AUGMENTATION

Although we try to both reduce the number of drugs we use in therapy and simplify the chemical makeup of those individual drugs in order to make them more efficient with fewer side effects, there are circumstances when it is appropriate to use two drugs together to treat certain situations. There are basically two reasons for using a combination (*augmentation*) of psychiatric medications: to treat multiple symptoms that cannot be treated successfully with a single medication or to aid the treatment of a single symptom that is not responding to a single medication. The following circumstances are four examples of drug combination use.

For example, I may have a patient who is suffering not only from depression but experiences occasional anxiety. I might begin by prescribing an antidepressant, such as DESYREL. However, if the DESYREL did not relieve the symptoms of anxiety along with the depression, I might prescribe an antianxiety drug, such as XANAX. The advantage of XANAX is that because it is short-acting, it should diminish or eliminate the anxiety but not stay in the body long enough to cause a possible additional drug interaction with the antidepressant.

A second example would be a patient who was experiencing massive mood changes, shifting from manic behavior and speech to depression. I might give this individual a major tranquilizer, such as HALDOL, PROLIXIN, or TRILAFON in combination with LITHIUM. The LITHIUM would act as a mood stabilizer but not treat the underlying psychosis; the underlying problem is the function of the other drugs, which are antipsychotic agents. Besides LITHIUM, some other drugs that can act as mood stabilizers in these cases are TEGRETOL, DEPAKOTE, or KLONOPIN.

A third circumstance also involves a psychotic drug. For example, if someone's depression were complicated by psychotic symptoms, such as profound shame, or the irrational fears of infidelity or a fatal illness, I might give this person an antipsychotic drug (these drugs are sometimes called *major tranquilizers*), such as HALDOL along with the antidepressant medication.

This sequence can be reversed: The patient might be recovering from a psychotic disorder, such as schizophrenia, and develop a depression. In this case, the patient might be given an antidepressant, in addition to the antipsychotic medication.

A fourth instance of combination use might be the case of someone whose depression is not responding to conventional antidepressants. If a patient has not received symptom relief after trying several antidepressants over a three-month period, then I would consider using LITHIUM with the antidepressant because it can augment or increase the effectiveness of the antidepressant drug. In the same regard, *psychostimulants* or *thyroid extracts* can be used to augment the effectiveness of an antidepressant, but these drugs are less preferable in that they introduce a greater number of possible side effects.

Brand Name	Generic Name
LIMBITROL, LIMBITROL-DS	chlordiazepoxide (klor-dye-az-e-POX-ide) and amitriptyline (a-mee-TRIP-ti-leen)

HOW THE DRUG WORKS

It is thought that this drug decreases the activity of the limbic area of the brain to reduce depression.

PURPOSE

Moderate to severe depression associated with moderate to severe anxiety.

DOSAGE

Treatment of depression and anxiety

Adults: (initially) three to four LIMBITROL tablets (they contain 10 mg chlordiazepoxide and 25 mg amitriptyline) daily, in divided doses, followed by two to six tablets daily as required.

SIDE EFFECTS

Common: Drowsiness; dizziness; dry mouth; blurred vision; constipation; weight gain; headache; bloating.

Uncommon: Diarrhea; nausea; vomiting; fatigue.

ADVERSE REACTIONS

Confusion; hallucinations; difficult urination; eye pain; depression; shakiness; insomnia; nervousness; irregular heartbeat. *Rare:* sensitivity to sunlight; seizures; sore throat and fever; skin rash; yellowing of eyes and skin.

DRUG INTERACTION

Increases the sedating effects of alcohol, sedative-hypnotics, and other CNS depressants, anticonvulsants, oral anticoagulants, and antihypertensive drugs.

With monoamine-oxidase (MAO) inhibitors, risk of extreme sedation, excitability, severe convulsions, coma, and death.

ANTABUSE and tricyclic antidepressants may increase effects of this drug.

OVERDOSAGE

If any of the following symptoms develops, notify your physician immediately: Rapid heartbeat; irregular heartbeat; congestive heart failure; muscle rigidity; convulsions; severe hypotension; stupor; coma.

Comments: LIMBITROL is considered a combination drug. It contains chlordiazepoxide and amitriptyline, which is LIBRIUM and ELAVAL. The drug is used for those individuals with depression who are significantly agitated or anxious. However, combination drugs, as such, are not commonly used because they increase the likelihood of side effects and adverse drug reactions. The basic aim of drug therapy is to work toward the use of only one drug and one with the cleanest or least likelihood of any side effects. For example, this drug must be used with caution by anyone who has had a history of urinary retention or glaucoma. Hence, these and other combination drugs are falling out of favor.

Pregnancy: Category D (see sidebar on page 69). This means that studies in pregnant women have shown a significant risk to the fetus. Therefore, the drug should be used only if needed in a serious disease and when other, safer drugs have proven to be ineffective or cannot be used.

ANTIPSYCHOTICS

The first antipsychotic drugs were developed in the late 1940s as part of a search for a drug that would provide presurgery patients with a calming effect without excessive sedation. In more recent years, research has revealed that the sedating or tranquilizing properties of these antipsychotic medications are directly related to the drug's ability to block one of the chemical messengers of the central nervous system: dopamine. By blocking the dopamine receptors in the brain, these antipsychotic drugs—also referred to as neuroleptic drugs or major tranquilizers—act to correct an imbalance of nerve impulse transmissions that appear to play some role in psychotic disorders.

Some of these drugs are also prescribed for the treatment of other ailments, such as Gilles de la Tourette's syndrome. On the other hand, none of them is the drug of choice for the treatment of short-term anxiety or insomnia. In general, they need to be used carefully, since they have potentially irreversible neuromuscular side effects, particularly when used over time.

Course of Treatment

The first goal of these drugs, especially when administered in rapid and frequent doses, is the relief of specific symptoms of psychosis, such as hostility, agitation, or combativeness. If the situation calls for immediate results, many of the drugs can be injected into the muscle, since the drug is more quickly absorbed in this form. Other symptoms of a psychotic illness, such as disordered thinking or abnormal suspicions, require longer treatment time.

It is important to understand that low doses are recommended for antipsychotic medications. To increase the dose does not increase their efficacy but does increase the likelihood of their side effects.

If the symptoms of agitation, distractibility, and insomnia persist after one or two weeks of drug therapy, your doctor will probably try some other family of medication. Your doctor may reduce medication to a once-a-day, often a nightly, schedule once your psychotic symptoms have been brought under control.

The treatment of psychotic symptoms with this type of medication usually has four stages:

1. For approximately a week you adjust to the presence of the drug; the drug produces no genuine therapeutic effects during this period.
2. From the second to the sixth week, you usually show some signs of improvement, both in terms of daily living skills and interpersonal relationships. At about this time, you should see improvements in symptoms of combativeness and hostility, followed by a general relief of tension and hyperactivity.
3. From this point on, the symptoms of delusions produced by the illness should be measurably diminished. Although the abnormal thoughts or ideas may occur at times during the course of the treatment, they are usually less intrusive; you should be able to lead a relatively normal life.
4. Once the symptoms are under basic control, you may be maintained on a low-dose regimen of an antipsychotic medication. Once the therapy has established a maintenance regimen of medication, the ongoing treatment may also include other forms of psychotherapy.

Potential Risks

The use of antipsychotic drugs poses potential risks for everyone, but some people are at greater risk than others.

Children   Many of the drugs in this family pose different risks for children. Some drugs shouldn't be used for children under the age of twelve; others can be given to children as young as six; and MELLARIL and HALDOL are occasionally given to children as young as three. In every instance of drug use, the weight, general health, and severity of the symptoms of the child are taken into consideration before any antipsychotic medication is prescribed.

Women   The safety of all these drugs for use during pregnancy has not been established. However, it is recommended that they can be used if the need is clear and the potential benefits to the mother outweigh the potential risks to the fetus. Speak to your physician about drug use during pregnancy. Also, if you intend to breast-feed, consult your doctor; two of these drugs, THORAZINE and HALDOL, are known to appear in breast milk. (See "Pregnant and Lactating Women," page 66.)

Elderly   Low doses of these drugs are both safer and sufficient for use among the elderly. People over the age of sixty are more susceptible to a variety of side effects, especially hypotension (low blood pressure) and tardive dyskinesia (involuntary and uncontrollable movements). Elderly women are especially vulnerable to tardive dyskinesia. Generally speaking, any increase or decrease in dosage should be made gradually, since changes can produce side effects or adverse reactions. (See "The Elderly," page 72.)

Withdrawal

Although antipsychotic drugs are not as dependent-liable (*addictive*) as are narcotics, if these drugs are abruptly stopped after long-term use or high-dose therapy, you could experience withdrawal symptoms such as headaches, nausea, dizziness, or an increased heart rate. These symptoms may begin within two to four days and last for as much as two weeks. In these instances, the symptoms can be reduced by gradually decreasing the dosage of the drug or by continuing with an anti-Parkinson drug for several weeks after the antipsychotic drug is withdrawn. (See "Antidyskinetics," page 227.)

Food-and-Drug Interactions

Avoid drinking alcohol with most, if not all, antipsychotic drugs since alcohol will enhance the effects of the drug; the drug will increase the intoxicating effect of the alcohol; and the combination will increase the risk of depression. An alkaline urine can prolong the effect of many of these drugs; hence, it is advised to avoid antacids that neutralize stomach acid because, by reducing the acid, they make the urine more alkaline.

Since THORAZINE, over time, will increase your body's need for vitamin B$_2$ (*riboflavin*), it is advised that you increase your vitamin B$_2$ intake. Milk is a good source, but a one-a-day multivitamin supplement is preferred since milk may increase the alkalinity of your urine.

Side Effects
The frequency and severity of side effects or adverse reactions depend on factors such as the strength of the dose, how long someone has taken the drug, and, of course, the susceptibility of the user. (See "People at Particular Risk," page 66.)

Physiological Effects of Antipsychotic Medications
Behavioral Restlessness, hyperactivity, confusion, depression, fear, hallucinations, severe fatigue.

Circulatory system Changes in blood pressure, light-headedness, or slow heart rate.

Dermatological Hives, rash, swelling, itching, red or dry skin, sensitivity to sunlight, hair loss (rare), flushing, sweating.

Digestive system Nausea, vomiting, loss or increase in appetite, constipation, diarrhea.

Head and eyes Sensitivity to light, blurred vision, glaucoma, nasal congestion.

Liver Yellowing of the skin or eyes (jaundice).

Muscular system Muscle spasms in the neck and back, rolling eyes, numbness in the legs and arms, tightness in the throat, difficulty swallowing (dysphagia), involuntary movement of the mouth, tongue, jaw, and face (see "Extrapyramidal Symptoms," page 39), muscle stiffness, rigidity, poor balance, shuffling walk.

Nervous system Headaches, fatigue, tremors, drooling, drowsiness, swelling of the brain (very rare), tardive dyskinesia (see page 292).

Respiratory system Difficulty swallowing or breathing, deeper breathing.

Guidelines for Use

Even though these drugs belong to the same family, they are not all necessarily equally effective, and they do not have the same side effects. You should never change from one drug to another without your doctor's permission.

If your medication ever causes you to vomit, see your doctor, since it may not be properly absorbed and, therefore, not effective.

Do not change the dosage of these drugs just because you think you may become dependent on it. If you think you have a problem, check with your doctor. A common side effect is drowsiness; hence avoid using any other medicines, such as OTC cold medicine, since they may increase the drowsiness. Also, use extreme caution while driving or using machinery that requires alertness or good coordination. Avoid sudden changes in position and use caution when climbing stairs, especially during the first week of therapy, as you may become quite dizzy. Exercise moderately in hot weather since these drugs increase your susceptibility to heat stroke.

Always call your doctor if the drug causes any side effects that persist for more than a week. Do not hesitate to notify your doctor if you experience involuntary muscle twitching, unusual bleeding or bruising, dark-colored urine and pale stools or other signs of jaundice, skin rash, impaired vision, sore throat, and fever.

ANTIPSYCHOTICS

LOW-POTENCY

Brand Name	Generic Name
THORAZINE	chlorpromazine (klor-PRO-ma-zeen)
MELLARIL, MILLAZINE	thioridazine (thye-oh-RID-a-zeen)
SERENTIL	mesoridazine (mez-o-RID-a-zeen)

HIGH-POTENCY

Brand Name	Generic Name
HALDOL	haloperidol (hey-lo-PAIR-ee-doll)
TRILAFON	perphenazine (per-FEN-a-zeen)
STELAZINE, SUPRAZINE	trifluoperazine (tri-FLOO-oh-pair-a-zeen)
NAVANE	thiothixene (thye-oh-THIX-een)
PROLIXIN, PERMITIL	fluphenazine (floo-FEN-a-zeen)
MOBAN	molindone (MO-lin-down)
LOXITANE	loxapine (LOX-a-peen)
COMPAZINE	prochlorperazine (pro-klor-PAIR-a-zeen)
ORAP	pimozide (PIM-oh-zide)
CLOZARIL	clozapine (KLAS-a-peen)

DEPOT

Brand Name	Generic Name
PROLIXIN	fluphenazine (floo-FEN-a-zeen) decanoate and fluphenazine enanthate
HALDOL	haloperidol (hey-lo-PAIR-ee-doll) decanoate
RISPERIDOL	risperidone (ris-PAIR-e-doan)

LOW-POTENCY

Brand Name	Generic Name
THORAZINE	chlorpromazine (klor-PRO-ma-zeen)

154

HOW THE DRUG WORKS

By blocking the dopamine receptors in the brain, this drug acts to correct an imbalance of nerve impulse transmissions that appear to play some role in psychotic disorders.

PURPOSE

Severe anxiety associated with psychotic disorders; also used to treat those symptoms associated with psychosis, such as delusions and hallucinations.

DOSAGE

Treatment of psychosis
  Adults: (mild) 25 mg to 100 mg; (moderate) 100 mg to 500 mg; (high) 500 mg to 1,000 mg (taken orally) in divided doses daily; 10 mg to 50 mg (injections), every one to four hours when needed.
  Children: Doses should never exceed 40 mg in children under five years or 75 mg in children aged five to twelve years.

SIDE EFFECTS

  Common: Drowsiness; dry mouth; constipation; urinary retention; skin rash; sensitivity to the sun.
  Uncommon: Tremors, muscle rigidity, and other symptoms similar to Parkinson's disease.

ADVERSE REACTIONS

Skin rash (due to allergic drug reaction); yellowing skin and eyes or dark urine, nausea, and vomiting (suggests drug-induced hepatitis); ejaculatory problems; impotence; tardive dyskinesia; neuroleptic malignant syndrome.

DRUG INTERACTION

Increases the effects of drugs such as alcohol and other CNS depressants; propanolol; anticholinergic.

Decreases the effects of drugs such as oral anticoagulants; centrally acting antihypertensive agents; lithium; barbiturates.

OVERDOSAGE

If any of the following symptoms develops, notify your physician immediately: Severe extrapyramidal symptoms (muscular weakness, rigidity, or tremors), depression, agitation, sleepiness, fever, convulsions, coma.

Comments: Because it is highly sedating, you should be very cautious about driving a car while taking THORAZINE: your reaction time will be severely impaired. When changing positions, such as getting up from a chair or rising from bed, move slowly or you may experience dizziness because of a sharp and unexpected drop in blood pressure.

If you intend to be in the sun, wear a sunscreen or protective clothing to avoid an easy sunburn and stay out of the sun during the hours of 11 A.M. to 2 P.M. since this is when the sun is most intense. Over time, this drug can raise blood cholesterol levels and increase your body's need for riboflavin (vitamin B_2). Do not drink alcohol while using this drug; reduce your consumption of dairy products as they cause alkaline urine levels to rise—which may cause the drug to remain longer in the body. For the same reason, do not use antacids less than two hours before or after taking this drug.

In a liquid form, the drug has a particularly sharp, unpleasant taste; if taken with fruit juice, however, it can be very palatable.

Pregnancy: Category C (see sidebar on page 69). This means that whatever risk the drug could conceivably pose for the fetus is outweighed by the possible benefits of the drug to the mother. However, you are advised to avoid its use during the first trimester of a pregnancy, whenever possible. Do not breast-feed with this drug because it appears in breast milk.

Brand Name
MELLARIL, MILLAZINE

Generic Name
thioridazine (thye-oh-RID-a-zeen)

HOW THE DRUG WORKS

By blocking the dopamine receptors in the brain, this drug acts to correct an imbalance of nerve impulse transmissions that appear to play some role in psychotic disorders.

PURPOSE

Severe anxiety associated with psychotic disorders; also used to treat those symptoms associated with psychosis, such as delusions and hallucinations; (because thought to have antidepressive qualities) given to people who have psychosis with depressive symptoms.

DOSAGE

Treatment of psychosis
   Adults: 25 to 400 mg (taken orally) in divided doses; under unusual circumstances, dosage can reach 800 mg daily in divided doses.
   Elderly (over age sixty-five): 10 to 50 mg (taken orally) in divided doses.

Treatment of symptoms of dementia in elderly
   Adults: initially, 25 mg (taken orally) in divided doses.

SIDE EFFECTS

   Common: Drowsiness; dry mouth; constipation; urinary retention.
   Uncommon: Neuroendocrine disorder; lactorrhea; amenorrhea; male breast enlargement; retrograde ejaculation.

ADVERSE REACTIONS

Tardive dyskinesia; neuroleptic malignant syndrome; retinopathy (impaired vision).

DRUG INTERACTION

Increases the effects of drugs such as alcohol and other CNS depressants.

Decreases the effects of drugs such as centrally acting antihypertensive agents; lithium; barbiturates.

OVERDOSAGE

If any of the following symptoms develops, notify your physician immediately: Severe extrapyramidal symptoms (muscular weakness, rigidity, or tremors), psychotic reactions, nausea, vomiting, hypotension, drowsiness.

Comments: MELLARIL is less sedating than THORAZINE (it doesn't make you so lethargic or dizzy) and it has fewer extrapyramidal side effects. On the other hand, the drug does not come in an injectable form. The upper dosage range of this drug is set at 800 mg; at higher levels it can cause a disorder of the retina which may affect your vision and cause permanent blindness. Tardive dyskinesia may occur with use over many months or years; neuroleptic malignant syndrome is also a health risk, but it is unrelated to how long the drug is used.

You should wear a sunscreen or protective clothing to avoid sunburn and stay out of the sun during the hours of 11 A.M. to 2 P.M., since this is when the sun is most intense. Do not drink alcohol with this drug and reduce your consumption of dairy products as they cause alkaline urine levels to rise, which may cause the drug to remain longer in the body. For the same reason, do not use antacids less than two hours before or after taking this drug.

Pregnancy: Category C (see sidebar on page 69). This means that whatever risk the drug could conceivably pose for the fetus is outweighed by the possible benefits of the drug to the mother. However, you are advised to avoid its use during the first trimester of a pregnancy, whenever possible.

Brand Name	*Generic Name*
SERENTIL	mesoridazine (mez-o-RID-a-zeen)

HOW THE DRUG WORKS

By blocking the dopamine receptors in the brain, this drug acts to correct an imbalance of nerve impulse transmissions that appear to play some role in psychotic disorders.

PURPOSE

Severe anxiety associated with psychotic disorders; also used to treat those symptoms associated with psychosis, such as delusions and hallucinations; (because thought to have antidepressive qualities) given to people who have psychosis with depressive symptoms.

DOSAGE

Treatment of anxiety associated with psychosis
Adults: 25 mg to 400 mg (taken orally) in divided doses; under unusual circumstances, dosage can reach 800 mg daily in divided doses.
Elderly (over age sixty-five): 10 mg to 50 mg (taken orally) in divided doses.

Treatment of symptoms of dementia in elderly
Adults: initially, 25 mg (taken orally) in divided doses.

SIDE EFFECTS

Common: Drowsiness; dry mouth; constipation; urinary retention.
Uncommon: Lactorrhea; male breast enlargement; retrograde ejaculation.

ADVERSE REACTIONS

Tardive dyskinesia; neuroleptic malignant syndrome; retinopathy (impaired vision).

DRUG INTERACTION

Increases the effects of drugs such as alcohol and other CNS depressants.

Decreases the effects of drugs such as centrally acting antihypertensive agents; lithium; barbiturates.

OVERDOSAGE

If any of the following symptoms develops, notify your physician immediately: Severe extrapyramidal symptoms (muscular weakness, rigidity, or tremors), depression, hypotension, drowsiness, convulsions, coma.

Comments: The lowest potency of all antipsychotic drugs, SERENTIL has the fewest of the anticholinergic side effects, such as dry mouth, is less sedating, and can be injected intramuscularly (in an emergency). The drug may cause some dizziness, but it is considered so mild that it is widely used in the treatment of the elderly and adolescents. You should wear a sunscreen or protective clothing to avoid sunburn and stay out of the sun during the hours of 11 A.M. to 2 P.M., since this is when the sun is most intense. If you are bothered by dry mouth, try sugarless gum or hard candy.

Pregnancy: Category C (see sidebar on page 69). This means that whatever risk the drug could conceivably pose for the fetus is outweighed by the possible benefits of the drug to the mother. However, you are advised to avoid its use during the first trimester of a pregnancy, whenever possible.

HIGH-POTENCY

These are high-potency dopamine blockers—five to twenty-five times more powerful than THORAZINE, MELLARIL, and SERENTIL. While these drugs have less sedation, hypotension, and relatively mild anticholinergic side effects, they are more likely to produce extrapyramidal symptoms or parkinsonian-like symptoms than the low-potency antipsychotic drugs.

Brand Name	*Generic Name*
HALDOL	haloperidol (hey-lo-PAIR-ee-doll)

HOW THE DRUG WORKS

By blocking the dopamine receptors in the brain, this drug acts to correct an imbalance of nerve impulse transmissions that appear to play some role in psychotic disorders.

PURPOSE

Severe anxiety associated with psychotic disorders; also used to treat those symptoms associated with psychosis, such as delusions and hallucinations; used in the treatment of Gilles de la Tourette's syndrome (tics and involuntary vocal utterances); in schizophrenia and manic-depressive illness; dementia in the elderly.

DOSAGE

Treatment of psychotic disorders
  Adults: (initially) 0.5 mg to 2 mg (taken orally) in divided doses; or (for severe chronic or resistant symptoms) 3 mg to 5 mg, followed by, if necessary, up to 100 mg daily. (See page 179 for HALOPERIDOL DECANOATE.)

Treatment of Gilles de la Tourette's syndrome
  Children: 2 mg to 20 mg (taken orally) in divided doses.

SIDE EFFECTS

  Common: Drowsiness; dry mouth; urinary retention.
  Uncommon: Muscle rigidity, tremors, and abnormal movements similar to Parkinson's disease.

ADVERSE REACTIONS

Tardive dyskinesia (e.g., chewing movements); impotence; neuroleptic malignant syndrome (rare).

DRUG INTERACTION

Increases the effects of drugs such as alcohol and other CNS depressants.

With LITHIUM in high doses, it may cause lethargy and confusion.

With METHYLDOPA, it may cause symptoms of dementia.

OVERDOSAGE

  If any of the following symptoms develops, notify your physician immediately: Severe extrapyramidal symptoms (muscular weakness, rigidity, or tremors), hypotension, drowsiness, coma.

Comments: A very powerful dopamine blocker, HALDOL is clinically twenty-five times more powerful than THORAZINE. It is a low-dose drug that causes little sedation, fewer anticholinergic side effects, or hypotension; therefore, it is effective in the elderly. It can be injected intramuscularly—useful if someone needs to be tranquilized quickly. (See page 179 for more information on the injected form of HALDOL.) It is perhaps the most commonly used major tranquilizer in hospitals. If you are bothered by dry mouth, try a sugarless gum or hard candy, but do not drink alcohol while taking this drug.

Pregnancy: Category C (see sidebar on page 69). This means that whatever risk the drug could conceivably pose for the fetus is outweighed by the possible benefits of the drug to the mother. However, you are advised to avoid its use during the first trimester of a pregnancy, whenever possible.

Brand Name	*Generic Name*
TRILAFON	perphenazine (per-FEN-a-zeen)

HOW THE DRUG WORKS

By blocking the dopamine receptors in the brain, this drug acts to correct an imbalance of nerve impulse transmissions that appear to play some role in psychotic disorders.

PURPOSE

Severe anxiety associated with psychotic disorders; also used to treat those symptoms associated with psychosis, such as delusions and hallucinations.

DOSAGE

Treatment of psychotic disorders

Adults: (dosage varies with each patient) 8 mg to 16 mg (taken orally) in divided doses; or 5 mg to 10 mg (injections) repeated as needed, every six hours, up to 15 mg daily for ambulatory patients and 30 mg for hospitalized patients.

Children: Use the lowest adult dosage.

SIDE EFFECTS

Common: Drowsiness; dry mouth; urinary retention; constipation.

Uncommon: Muscle rigidity, tremors, and abnormal movements similar to Parkinson's disease.

ADVERSE REACTIONS

Tardive dyskinesia (e.g., chewing movements); neuroleptic malignant syndrome (rare); severe, acute hypotension.

DRUG INTERACTION

Increases the effects of drugs such as alcohol and other CNS depressants.

With barbiturates, may decrease effectiveness of drug.

OVERDOSAGE

If any of the following symptoms develops, notify your physician immediately: Severe extrapyramidal symptoms, nausea, vomiting, difficulty swallowing.

Comments: At low doses, TRILAFON has relatively lower incidence of anticholinergic side effects than other high-potency antipsychotic drugs; any drowsiness and dizziness should cease after the first two weeks. It is so well tolerated by patients that it seems to be popular now as a replacement for the harsher experience of HALDOL. It can be injected intramuscularly if someone needs to be tranquilized quickly. Do not drink alcohol while taking this drug and do not take antacids two hours before or after taking the drug. If you are in the sun, wear a sunscreen or protective clothing to avoid sunburn, and stay out of the sun during the hours of 11 A.M. to 2 P.M., since this is when the sun is most intense.

Pregnancy: Category C (see sidebar on page 69). This means that whatever risk the drug could conceivably pose for the fetus is outweighed by the possible benefits of the drug to the mother. However,

you are advised to avoid its use during the first trimester of a pregnancy, whenever possible. _____

Brand Name	*Generic Name*
STELAZINE,	trifluoperazine (tri-
SUPRAZINE	FLOO-oh-pair-
	a-zeen)

HOW THE DRUG WORKS

By blocking the dopamine receptors in the brain, this drug acts to correct an imbalance of nerve impulse transmissions that appear to have some role in psychotic disorders.

PURPOSE

Severe anxiety associated with psychotic disorders; also used to treat those symptoms associated with psychosis, such as delusions and hallucinations; also used to treat anxiety, but is not the drug of choice.

DOSAGE

Treatment of psychotic disorders
   Adults: (dosage varies with each patient) 2 mg to 5 mg (taken orally) in divided doses, up to 40 mg; usual maintenance dosage: 15 mg to 20 mg.
   Children (six through thirteen years): (closely supervised) initially, 1 mg, up to 15 mg for older children.

Treatment of nonpsychotic anxiety
   Adults: 1 mg to 2 mg (taken orally), not to exceed 6 mg for more than twelve weeks.

SIDE EFFECTS

   Common: Drowsiness; dry mouth; urinary retention.
   Uncommon: Muscle rigidity, tremors, and abnormal movements similar to Parkinson's disease; constipation.

ADVERSE REACTIONS

Tardive dyskinesia (e.g., chewing movements); neuroleptic malignant syndrome (rare).

DRUG INTERACTION

Increases the effects of drugs such as alcohol and other CNS depressants.

With barbiturates or LITHIUM, it may decrease the effectiveness of the drug.

With antihypertensives, it decreases their effects.

OVERDOSAGE

If any of the following symptoms develops, notify your physician immediately: Depression, severe weakness, hypotension, agitation, convulsions, fever.

Comments: One of the older of the high-potency major tranquilizers, STELAZINE is used intramuscularly if someone needs to be tranquilized quickly. For many years it was given to people taking THORAZINE to reduce that drug's orthostatic hypotension and sedating effects. However, those combinations of major tranquilizers are not used today because of the increased risk of adverse reactions. Instead, someone today is often given HALDOL or TRILAFON.

Any drowsiness and dizziness from this drug should cease after the first two weeks. Change positions slowly to avoid sudden dizziness. Do not drink alcohol while taking this drug or take antacids two hours before or after taking this drug. If you are in the sun, wear a sunscreen or protective clothing to avoid sunburn, and stay out of the sun during the hours of 11 A.M. to 2 P.M., since this is when the sun is most intense.

Pregnancy: Category C (see sidebar on page 69). This means that whatever risk the drug could conceivably pose for the fetus is outweighed by the possible benefits of the drug to the mother. However, you are advised to avoid its use during the first trimester of a pregnancy, whenever possible.

Brand Name	Generic Name
NAVANE	thiothixene (thye-oh-THIX-een)

HOW THE DRUG WORKS

By blocking the dopamine receptors in the brain, this drug acts to correct an imbalance of nerve impulse transmissions that appear to have some role in psychotic disorders.

PURPOSE

Severe anxiety associated with psychotic disorders; also used to treat those symptoms associated with psychosis, such as delusions and hallucinations.

DOSAGE

Treatment of psychotic disorders

Adults: initially, 2 mg (taken orally) in divided doses, to 15 mg (usual maintenance dosage 20 mg to 30 mg); some patients can be maintained on single daily doses. If started on injection, 4 mg dosage up to 30 mg; however, patient should be changed to oral medication as soon as possible.

SIDE EFFECTS

Common: Drowsiness; dry mouth; urinary retention; increased appetite; nasal congestion; lactorrhea.

Uncommon: Muscle rigidity, tremors, and abnormal movements similar to Parkinson's disease; constipation.

ADVERSE REACTIONS

Tardive dyskinesia (e.g., chewing movements); neuroleptic malignant syndrome (rare); paradoxical exacerbation of psychotic symptoms. (See "Adverse Reactions," page 37.)

DRUG INTERACTION

Increases the effects of drugs such as alcohol and other CNS depressants.

OVERDOSAGE

If any of the following symptoms develops, notify your physician immediately: Muscular twitching, depression, severe weakness, drooling, agitation, convulsions, fever, coma.

Comments: NAVANE is a low-sedating drug with a relatively low incidence of anticholinergic and cardiovascular side effects. It has become more popular recently because its usual side effects are relatively mild.

Any drowsiness and dizziness from the drug should cease after the first two weeks. Change positions slowly to avoid sudden dizziness due to hypotension. The drug can be injected intramuscularly if someone needs to be tranquilized quickly. Do not drink alcohol while taking this drug. If you are in the sun, wear a sunscreen or protective clothing to avoid sunburn. Also, stay out of the sun during the hours of 11 A.M. to 2 P.M. since this is when the sun is most intense.

Pregnancy: Category C (see sidebar on page 69). This means that whatever risk the drug could conceivably pose for the fetus is outweighed by the possible benefits of the drug to the mother. However, you are advised to avoid its use during the first trimester of a pregnancy, whenever possible.

Brand Name	*Generic Name*
PROLIXIN, PERMITIL	fluphenazine (floo-FEN-a-zeen)

HOW THE DRUG WORKS

By blocking the dopamine receptors in the brain, this drug acts to correct an imbalance of nerve impulse transmissions that appear to have some role in psychotic disorders.

PURPOSE

Severe anxiety associated with psychotic disorders; also used to treat those symptoms associated with psychosis, such as delusions and hallucinations.

DOSAGE

Treatment of psychotic disorders

Adults: initially, 2.5 mg to 10.0 mg (taken orally) in divided doses, every six to eight hours, up to 20 mg daily, if needed; 1 mg to 5 mg is the usual maintenance dosage.

Children: 2.5 mg to 3.5 mg daily in divided doses; maximum dose should be no more than 10 mg.

SIDE EFFECTS

Common: Drowsiness; dry mouth; urinary retention; increased appetite; nasal congestion; lactorrhea.

Uncommon: Muscle rigidity, tremors, and abnormal movements similar to Parkinson's disease; constipation.

ADVERSE REACTIONS

Uncommon: Tardive dyskinesia (e.g., chewing movements); neuroleptic malignant syndrome (rare); convulsions.

DRUG INTERACTION

Increases the effects of drugs such as alcohol and other CNS depressants.

With barbiturates and lithium, may decrease effectiveness of drug.

With antihypertensives, it decreases antihypertensive effects.

OVERDOSAGE

If any of the following symptoms develops, notify your physician immediately: Muscular twitching or rigidity, depression, severe weakness, blurred vision, severe hypotension, agitation.

Comments: PROLIXIN is a low-sedating drug with a high incidence of extrapyramidal symptoms, such as muscle spasms, severe stiffness, and rolling of the eyes. It also comes in a long-acting injectable form known as PROLIXIN DECANOATE (see page 177), which makes it easier to establish a steady-state blood level. This form of the drug may produce more side effects or adverse reactions.

Any drowsiness and dizziness from this drug should cease after the first two weeks. Change positions slowly to avoid sudden dizziness. Do not take antacids two hours before or after taking this drug and do not drink alcohol. If you are in the sun, wear a sunscreen or protective clothing to avoid sunburn, and stay out of the sun during the hours of 11 A.M. to 2 P.M., since this is when the sun is most intense.

Pregnancy: Category C (see sidebar on page 69). This means that whatever risk the drug could conceivably pose for the fetus is outweighed by the possible benefits of the drug to the mother. However, you are advised to avoid its use during the first trimester of a pregnancy, whenever possible.

Brand Name	*Generic Name*
MOBAN	molindone (MO-lin-down)

HOW THE DRUG WORKS

By blocking the dopamine receptors in the brain, this drug acts to correct an imbalance of nerve impulse transmissions that appear to have some role in psychotic disorders.

PURPOSE

Severe anxiety associated with psychotic disorders; also used to treat those symptoms associated with psychosis, such as delusions and hallucinations.

DOSAGE

Treatment of psychotic disorders
Adults: (builds gradually) initially, 50 mg to 75 mg (taken orally) in divided doses; increased in three to four days to 100 mg daily, then, if necessary, up to 225 mg daily; (depending upon conditions) maintenance is 5 mg to 15 mg three or four times daily (mild), 10 mg to 25 mg three or four times daily (moderate).

SIDE EFFECTS

Common: Drowsiness; dry mouth; urinary retention; nasal congestion.

Uncommon: Muscle rigidity, tremors, and abnormal movements similar to Parkinson's disease; decreased sexual ability.

ADVERSE REACTIONS

Tardive dyskinesia (e.g., chewing movements); neuroleptic malignant syndrome (rare); convulsions.

DRUG INTERACTION

Increases the effects of drugs such as alcohol and other CNS depressants.

OVERDOSAGE

If any of the following symptoms develops, notify your physician immediately: Muscular twitching or rigidity, depression, severe weakness, blurred vision, seizures, agitation.

Comments: A low-sedating drug, MOBAN may require higher doses than are indicated in the guidelines. The drug appears to have a low incidence of extrapyramidal symptoms, such as muscle spasms, severe stiffness, and rolling of the eyes, and it may be effective in patients suffering from tardive dyskinesia. It can also be given in a single daily dose once effective levels have been established.

Any drowsiness and dizziness from the drug should cease after the first two weeks. Change positions slowly to avoid sudden dizziness, and do not drink alcohol with this drug. Dry mouth can be relieved with sugarless gum or hard candy.

Pregnancy: Category C (see sidebar on page 69). This means that whatever risk the drug could conceivably pose for the fetus is outweighed by the possible benefits of the drug to the mother. However, you are advised to avoid its use during the first trimester of a pregnancy, whenever possible.

Brand Name
LOXITANE

Generic Name
loxapine (LOX-a-peen)

HOW THE DRUG WORKS

By blocking the dopamine receptors in the brain, this drug acts to correct an imbalance of nerve impulse transmissions that appear to have some role in psychotic disorders.

PURPOSE

Severe anxiety associated with psychotic disorders; also used to treat those symptoms associated with psychosis, such as delusions and hallucinations.

DOSAGE

Treatment of psychotic disorders
   Adults: (doses vary) initially, 10 mg (taken orally) in divided doses, but rapidly increased over seven to ten days up to a maximum of 250 mg daily, until symptoms abate. Usual dosage is 60 mg to 100 mg daily in divided doses.

SIDE EFFECTS

   Common: Drowsiness; dry mouth; confusion; menstrual irregularity.
   Uncommon: Lactorrhea; male and female breast enlargement; muscle rigidity, tremors, and abnormal movements similar to Parkinson's disease.

ADVERSE REACTIONS

Tardive dyskinesia (e.g., chewing movements); neuroleptic malignant syndrome (rare); yellowing skin and eyes or dark urine (suggests drug-induced hepatitis); difficulty in speaking or swallowing.

DRUG INTERACTION

Increases the effects of drugs such as alcohol and other CNS depressants.

OVERDOSAGE

If any of the following symptoms develops, notify your physician immediately: (Depending upon dosage) from convulsions and severe hypotension to respiratory collapse and unconsciousness.

Comments: A moderately sedating drug, LOXITANE is sometimes used with antidepressants for people with psychotic depression who are not agitated, that is, people who need not be sedated. It is often given in a concentrate or liquid form, LOXITANE C (loxapine hydrochloride), usually mixed with fruit juice.

Weight gain and an increased appetite are two distracting side effects of this drug. Any drowsiness and dizziness from the drug should cease after the first two weeks; however, change positions slowly to avoid sudden dizziness due to hypotension. Dry mouth can be relieved with sugarless gum or hard candy.

Pregnancy: Category C (see sidebar on page 69). This means that whatever risk the drug could conceivably pose for the fetus is outweighed by the possible benefits of the drug to the mother. However, you are advised to avoid its use during the first trimester of a pregnancy, whenever possible.

Brand Name	*Generic Name*
COMPAZINE	prochlorperazine (pro-klor-PAIR-a-zeen)

HOW THE DRUG WORKS

By blocking the dopamine receptors in the brain, this drug acts to correct an imbalance of nerve impulse transmissions that appear to have some role in psychotic disorders. By blocking another chemical, acetylcholine (which transmits nerve impulses), the drug depresses stimulation of the vomiting center.

PURPOSE

Severe anxiety associated with psychotic disorders; relief of severe nausea and vomiting; not the drug of choice for short-term anxiety.

DOSAGE

Treatment of psychotic disorders

Adults: (for mild conditions) 5 mg to 10 mg (taken orally) in divided doses; (for immediate control of severe conditions) 10 mg to 20 mg (injections) and may be repeated every one to four hours until symptoms are controlled, then switch to oral form.

Children two to twelve years: initially, 2.5 mg to 10 mg (taken orally or rectally), not to exceed 20 mg daily for children two to five years, and 25 mg for children six to twelve years.

SIDE EFFECTS

Common: Drowsiness; dry mouth; confusion; menstrual irregularity.

Uncommon: Lactorrhea; male and female breast enlargement; muscle rigidity; tremors and abnormal movements similar to Parkinson's disease.

ADVERSE REACTIONS

Tardive dyskinesia (e.g., chewing movements); neuroleptic malignant syndrome (rare); oculogyric crisis; yellowing skin and eyes or dark urine (suggests drug-induced hepatitis); difficulty in speaking or swallowing.

DRUG INTERACTION

Increases the effects of all sedatives, sleep-inducing drugs, tranquilizers, antihistamines.

Decreases the effects of antiparkinson medications (e.g., levodopa).

With antidepressants, it may increase the effectiveness of the drug.

OVERDOSAGE

If any of the following symptoms develops, notify your physician immediately: Depression, extreme weakness, sleepiness, hypotension, muscle spasms, restlessness, agitation, fever, convulsions, coma.

Comments: Better known as a drug to control severe nausea or vomiting, COMPAZINE is used frequently for preoperative patients. It is also effective for the treatment of anxiety, tension, and agitation in people suffering from a psychotic disorder.

The elderly should receive only the lower range of dosages as it is highly sedating. Its concentrated form can be given with other liquids, such as fruit juice, coffee and tea, carbonated beverages, and soups.

Pregnancy: Category C (see sidebar on page 69). This means that whatever risk the drug could conceivably pose for the fetus is outweighed by the possible benefits of the drug to the mother. However, you are advised to avoid its use during the first trimester of a pregnancy, whenever possible.

Brand Name	*Generic Name*
ORAP	pimozide (PIM-oh-zide)

HOW THE DRUG WORKS

By blocking the dopamine receptors in the brain, this drug acts to correct an imbalance of nerve impulse transmissions that appear to have some role in psychotic disorders.

PURPOSE

Severe motor and phonic tics (twitching and involuntary vocal utterances) associated with Gilles de la Tourette's syndrome.

DOSAGE

Treatment of Gilles de la Tourette's disorder
Adults: initially, 1 mg to 2 mg (taken orally) daily in divided doses; increase dosages every other day. Maintenance dosage up to 10 mg daily.

SIDE EFFECTS

Common: Drowsiness; dry mouth; constipation, blurred vision, light-headedness.
Uncommon: Muscle rigidity, tremors, and abnormal movements similar to Parkinson's disease.

ADVERSE REACTIONS

Tardive dyskinesia (e.g., chewing movements); neuroleptic malignant syndrome (rare); difficulty in speaking or swallowing; rapid heartbeat; irregular blood pressure; restlessness; decreased sexual ability.

DRUG INTERACTION

Increases the effects of drugs such as alcohol and other CNS depressants.

With phenothiazine (e.g., chlorpromazine) and tricyclic antidepressants, the drug increases risk of ECG abnormalities.

OVERDOSAGE

If any of the following symptoms develops, notify your physician immediately: Depression, extreme weakness, hypotension, muscle spasms, restlessness, agitation, fever, seizures, coma.

Comments: Highly effective for those people who have Gilles de la Tourette's syndrome, ORAP is recommended if HALDOL has not been effective. Because it has serious side effects, ORAP (and CLOZARIL) is generally not prescribed unless the patient has failed to respond to standard treatment. ORAP has a high cardiovascular toxicity, that is, it can cause abnormal heart rhythms, sharp changes in blood pressure, and heart palpitations. Ten percent of the people who take the drug are later found to have electrocardiographic abnormalities. For these reasons, people should be carefully monitored by electrocardiogram and prescribed dosages should not be exceeded. Finally, the drug should not be stopped abruptly; when discontinued, it should be tapered.

Pregnancy: Category C (see sidebar on page 69). This means that whatever risk the drug could conceivably pose for the fetus is outweighed by the possible benefits of the drug to the mother. However, you are advised to avoid its use during the first trimester of a pregnancy, whenever possible.

Brand Name	*Generic Name*
CLOZARIL	clozapine (KLAS-a-peen)

HOW THE DRUG WORKS

By blocking the dopamine receptors in the brain, this drug acts to correct an imbalance of nerve impulse transmissions that appear to have some role in psychotic disorders.

PURPOSE

Chronic *treatment-resistant* schizophrenia; treatment of tardive dyskinesia.

DOSAGE

Treatment of tardive dyskinesia, schizophrenia
   Adults: (initially) 25 mg to 50 mg (taken orally) daily; increase dosages 25 mg to 50 mg daily to target dose of 300 mg to 450 mg daily.

SIDE EFFECTS

Common: Drowsiness; watery mouth; constipation; weight gain. *Uncommon:* Extrapyramidal side effects.

ADVERSE REACTIONS

Rapid heartbeat; hypotension; hypertension; fever. *Rare:* seizures (dose-related); agranulocytosis.

DRUG INTERACTION

It should be used with caution with other CNS medicines or protein-bound drugs, such as digoxin. It may increase the potency of anti-depressant medications. With PROZAC it may cause an increase in the side effects of CLOZARIL and produce bradycardia, or a slow heartbeat.

OVERDOSAGE

If any of the following symptoms develops, notify your physician immediately: Altered state of consciousness; drowsiness; hypotension; respiratory depression; seizures; delirium; coma.

Comments: Considered the first new drug (1989) to be marketed for the treatment of schizophrenia in about twenty years, CLOZAPINE is thought to be effective in patients who do not respond to the conventional major tranquilizers. It is also used because it alleges to have a low incidence of extrapyramidal symptoms, such as tremors, muscular rigidity, or uncoordinated movements, and a low incidence of tardive dyskinesia, a potentially irreversible condition with symptoms such as involuntary movements of the mouth, face, arms, and legs. The drug is thought to be especially effective in the treatment of so-called negative symptoms, such as social withdrawal, blunted feeling (the same low affect in response to different feeling states), or lack of spontaneity.

On the other hand, this drug causes a profound decrease in the body's ability to create white blood cells (*agranulocytosis*). However, if agranulocytosis (see page 287) should occur with the use of CLOZA-RIL, the risk decreases after six months of use and is negligible after the first year. Cautionary procedures call for weekly monitoring of blood samples, which can be performed by a team in your home. Needless to say, this is a very expensive procedure and is used only in those individuals for whom all other drugs have proved to be ineffective.

Pregnancy: Category B (see sidebar on page 69). This means the risk to the fetus is relatively low.

DEPOT

These antipsychotic drugs are injected or deposited (*depot* means *deposit* or *store*) deep into the muscle and, since they have a slow, consistent release, they need to be administered at intervals of only once a week to twice a month. These predominately long-acting drugs are prescribed for people who are noncompliant or reluctant to take the other major tranquilizers, but who clearly have multiple and recurring psychotic episodes that would require a maintenance medication. Intramuscular injections of these drugs are also indicated for people who are unable to metabolize major tranquilizers in an oral form.

Brand Name	*Generic Name*
PROLIXIN	fluphenazine (floo-FEN-a-zeen) decanoate and fluphenazine enanthate

HOW THE DRUG WORKS

By blocking the dopamine receptors in the brain, this drug acts to correct an imbalance of nerve impulse transmissions that appear to have some role in psychotic disorders.

PURPOSE

Severe anxiety associated with psychotic disorders; for people requiring prolonged antipsychotic drug therapy.

DOSAGE

Treatment of psychotic disorders
DECANOATE
   Adults: initially, 12.5 mg to 25 mg (injections); dosage can gradually be increased to 100 mg.
ENANTHATE
   Adults: initially, 25 mg every 2 weeks; dosages up to 100 mg; in doses above 50 mg, blood levels will be closely monitored.

SIDE EFFECTS

   Common: Drowsiness; dry mouth; urinary retention; increased appetite; nasal congestion; lactorrhea.
   Uncommon: Muscle rigidity, tremors, and abnormal movements similar to Parkinson's disease; constipation.

ADVERSE REACTIONS

Tardive dyskinesia (e.g., chewing movements); neuroleptic malignant syndrome (rare); convulsions.

DRUG INTERACTION

Increases the effects of drugs such as alcohol and other CNS depressants.

With barbiturates and lithium, it may decrease the effectiveness of the drug.

With antihypertensives, it decreases their effects.

OVERDOSAGE

If any of the following symptoms develops, notify your physician immediately: Muscular twitching or rigidity, depression, severe weakness, blurred vision, severe hypotension, agitation.

Comments: The major forms of depot medications are fluphenazine decanoate and fluphenazine enanthate, although the former is more popular. The decanoate form causes prolonged steady release of the drug and, therefore, produces a steady-state blood level over a period of as long as two weeks. In some instances, an injection may be effective for as long as four weeks. The length of time needed to establish an adequate blood level varies; but frequently, it takes up to three weeks.

Initially, injections are given on a weekly basis; but the nature of the action of the drug is such that it may accumulate in the body. Consequently, after three or four weeks the interval between the injections has to be increased or the dosage decreased. Some physicians will use both the oral dose, taken in daily divided doses, together with a weekly injection for the first three weeks; then, they will drop the oral dose.

Pregnancy: Category C (see sidebar on page 69). This means that whatever risk the drug could conceivably pose for the fetus is outweighed by the possible benefits of the drug to the mother. However, you are advised to avoid its use during the first trimester of a pregnancy, whenever possible.

Brand Name	*Generic Name*
HALDOL	haloperidol (hey-lo-PAIR-ee-doll) decanoate

HOW THE DRUG WORKS

By blocking the dopamine receptors in the brain, this drug acts to correct an imbalance of nerve impulse transmissions that appear to have some role in psychotic disorders.

PURPOSE

Severe anxiety associated with psychotic disorders, for people requiring prolonged antipsychotic drug therapy.

DOSAGE

Treatment of psychotic disorders

Adults: 50 mg to 100 mg (injections) every four weeks; the intervals between doses is about four weeks.

SIDE EFFECTS

Common: Drowsiness; dry mouth; urinary retention.

Uncommon: Muscle rigidity, tremors, and abnormal movements similar to Parkinson's disease.

ADVERSE REACTIONS

Tardive dyskinesia (e.g., chewing movements); neuroleptic malignant syndrome (rare).

DRUG INTERACTION

Increases the effects of drugs such as alcohol and other CNS depressants.

With lithium in high doses, it may cause lethargy and confusion.

With METHYLDOPA, it may cause symptoms of dementia.

OVERDOSAGE

If any of the following symptoms develops, notify your physician immediately: Severe extrapyramidal symptoms (e.g., muscular weakness, rigidity, or tremors), hypotension, drowsiness, coma.

Comments: A second form of depot drug is haloperidol decanoate. Often the patient is given daily doses of the oral form of HALDOL (see page 160) and then, converted by a factor multiplied by ten to fifteen times the oral dose, is given a single intramuscular dose of this drug on a monthly basis. In some cases, the factor may be twenty times the daily oral dose; there has been some difficulty achieving effective doses.

Pregnancy: Category C (see sidebar on page 69). This means that whatever risk the drug could conceivably pose for the fetus is outweighed by the possible benefits of the drug to the mother. However, you are advised to avoid its use during the first trimester of a pregnancy, whenever possible.

Brand Name	Generic Name
RISPERIDOL	risperidone (ris-PAIR-e-doan)

HOW THE DRUG WORKS

By blocking specific dopamine and serotonin receptor sites.

PURPOSE

Treatment of acute and chronic schizophrenia, aggressive behavior, and Gilles de la Tourette's syndrome.

DOSAGE

Adults: (Initially) 1 mg twice a day; doses can be titrated to 2 mg twice a day. RISPERIDOL originally had a maximum dose of 8 mg per day, but, in some instances, doses up to 20 mg have been used on an in-patient basis.

SIDE EFFECTS

Common: Insomnia; agitation; anxiety; fatigue; headache; weight gain; increased dreaming.
Uncommon: Hypotension (low blood pressure); back pain; irritated sinus; dandruff; diminished sexual desire.

ADVERSE REACTIONS

The incidence of extrapyramidal symptoms (eps) is very low when using small doses of the medication. As the dosage is raised above 6 mg per day, neuromuscular symptoms (eps) are similar to those of other high-potency antipsychotics. Recently, the first case of tardive dyskinesia has been described with symptoms such as chewing movements, but this possibly irreversible side effect does remain rare. Like other high-potency antipsychotic agents, this drug may lead to neuroleptic malignant syndrome with symptoms such as severe muscle rigidity, fever, and high blood pressure. Remedial treatment must be initiated immediately at first sign of these threatening disorders.

DRUG INTERACTION

Decreases the effects of levodopa.

When taken with carbamazepine (TEGRETOL), it will decrease the effect of this drug.

When taken with clozapine (CLOZARIL), it may increase the effects of this drug.

Do not take with alcohol or antihypertensive drugs, as it may enhance their depressant effects.

OVERDOSAGE

If any of the following symptoms develop, notify your physician immediately: Drowsiness; excessive fatigue; muscle stiffness; rapid heartbeat or irregular pulse; high or low blood pressure; and seizures.

Comments: Introduced late in 1993, RISPERIDOL is an increasingly popular antipsychotic drug because it generally produces few side effects. It is effective against positive symptoms such as hallucinations and delusions and is thought to be effective against negative symptoms, such as social withdrawal, blunting of feelings, and lack of spontaneous actions or speech.

Recently the drug was found to have antidepressant effects, which is meaningful, since depression often accompanies psychoses. Although not recommended at this time, the drug has been used experimentally to treat children with pervasive developmental disorder, formerly known as childhood autism.

The drug should not be used in patients with mood cycles because it can trigger a manic episode. On some occasions, a drop in orthostatic hypotension can cause dizziness when rising to a standing position. RISPERIDOL may cause increased prolactin levels that may result in abnormal menses and a tenderness and discharge in both male and female breasts.

Pregnancy: Category B (see sidebar on page 69). This means that the risk to the fetus is assumed to be relatively low. The effects of this drug during pregnancy, however, have not been studied. Hence, notify your doctor if you plan to become pregnant.

GATEWAY DRUGS

We have discovered much about brain function in recent years, but this remarkable organ still remains largely *terra incognita*. REVIA (naltrexone) (see page 185) and COGNEX (tacrine) (see page 187) are two medications that act as probes into areas of the brain about which we have only a limited understanding: the little-known opiate system and the neurotransmitters that connect the complex system of thought and memory. The two drugs deal with two illnesses, alcoholism and Alzheimer's disease, two chronic and progressive conditions with devastating effects on individuals and their families and enormous cost to our health-care system. What's noteworthy is that these two medications have opened new areas of research and development in their application of psychopharmacology to illnesses that have been somewhat peripheral to mainstream psychiatric disorders and that have had only a limited history of responding successfully to drug treatment.

The breakthrough in our understanding more about the opiate system started in the early 1970s, during a time of an incipient heroin epidemic in this country. As often happens in the world of research, the discovery of the opiate receptor was made simultaneously, in this instance by scientists working in New York, Palo Alto, Baltimore, and Scotland. The researchers learned that there are at least three opiate receptors and each has its own neurotransmitter or messenger. The receptors were named *mu*, *kappa*, and *sigma*. Stimulating the *mu* receptors, the site for all of our common analgesics, produced euphoria, or a keen sense of well-being; the *kappa* receptors caused quite the opposite effect, or dysphoria. And stimulation of the *sigma* receptors, to which the commonly abused drug PCP, or angel dust, binds, appeared to cause psychosis. We have yet to harness this particular receptor, but its identification suggests that one day we may develop an effective treatment for terribly incapacitating illnesses.

REVIA is used as an adjunctive treatment for alcohol dependence and is the first new treatment for alcoholism in forty-five years since the introduction of ANTABUSE. By blocking the *mu* receptor, REVIA denies the patient the "high" usually associated with alcohol. The net effect is to reduce craving and, thus, decrease the consumption of alcohol, reinforcing sobriety.

COGNEX involves the neurotransmitter acetylcholine. Researchers in choline chemistry had established some years ago that choline affected the function of memory. Their problem was how to provide more choline and, most important, to make sure it could breach the blood's brain barrier in order to be effective. The first product, a precursor of acetylcholine, seemed to work but it tasted bad and caused the patient to smell like fish. A second product, lecithin, required huge amounts as medication and had to be taken in shakes and malteds. Today, patients have available to them a much easier and far more effective product: the drug COGNEX, or tacrine. By blocking the natural breakdown of acetylcholine, the medication is able to provide an increased amount of this neurotransmitter, which acts on the cognitive areas of the frontal lobes that influence memory. For those who tolerate COGNEX, it provides an objective improvement in their memory and psychosocial functioning.

It should be noted that these drugs do not resolve the underlying problem but only delay the progression of the illness. They act as holding agents rather than as curative ones. Thus, like other psychotropic drugs, they must be used in conjunction with other supportive services in a comprehensive program of rehabilitation that, to be effective, must sometimes continue for the life of the patient.

GATEWAY DRUGS

ANTI-CRAVING AGENT

Brand Name   *Generic Name*
REVIA   naltrexone (nal-TRECKS-zone)

COGNITIVE ENHANCEMENT AGENT

Brand Name   *Generic Name*
COGNEX   tacrine (TA-kreen)

ANTI-CRAVING AGENT

Brand Name   *Generic Name*
REVIA   naltrexone (nal-TRECKS-zone)

HOW THE DRUG WORKS

By binding to opiate receptors and blocking the natural opiate system, a complex system of nerve centers and neurotransmitters governing the modulation of pain and perhaps many other regulatory systems, the drug reverses the intoxicating effects, or high, associated with alcohol and many other narcotic drugs and reduces craving.

PURPOSE

Treatment of narcotic and alcohol addiction.

DOSAGE

Treatment of alcoholism
Adults: 50 mg daily (taken orally), or a maximum total of 350 mg per week in two or three divided doses.
Elderly: Smaller doses for shorter periods.

Treatment of narcotic addiction
Adults: (A flexible approach to dosing may be employed) 50 mg every day (taken orally) and 100 mg on Saturday with a maximum total of 350 mg per week; or 100 mg every other day and 150 mg every third day (schedule: 100 mg Monday, 100 mg Wednesday, and 150 mg Friday). It may be recommended that half doses be prescribed

initially to assure an opiate dependent individual does not experience signs of withdrawal.

SIDE EFFECTS

Common: Nausea; headaches; dizziness; nervousness; insomnia; fatigue; muscle pain; vomiting; constipation; increased thirst; decreased appetite.

Uncommon: Diarrhea; abdominal pain; blurred vision; confusion; rash; earache.

Rare: Ringing in the ear; difficulty with ejaculation; impotence; pain and tenderness in the feet.

ADVERSE REACTIONS

Tremors; sweating; shaking; runny nose; watery eyes or tearing; rapid pulse.

DRUG INTERACTION

Decreases the effects of narcotic medications, including codeine, and can cause withdrawal symptoms.

If taken with isoniazid, can increase risk of liver damage.

OVERDOSAGE

If any of the following symptoms develop, notify your physician immediately: Rapid heartbeat; fainting; breathing difficulties; seizures; coma.

Comments: Naltrexone has been used for more than a decade in the treatment of narcotic addicts, under the brand name TREXAN. The same drug, used at lower dosages, has been found to reduce the high of alcohol and reduce cravings. Thus, naltrexone is being marketed under the brand name of REVIA for this use. It is also being studied in the treatment of childhood autism and eating and sleeping disorders.

The intent of the individual is important if the drug is to be helpful. Namely, it is usually effective in those individuals who have chosen sobriety and among those with the most to lose if their addictive behavior were to continue. The use of medication, such as REVIA, should be considered only one of many factors determining the success of treatment, such as the type, intensity, and duration of support treatment. Treatment with naltrexone should not be attempted in treatment of narcotic addiction unless the individual has remained opioid-free for at least a week or more.

This drug is not thought to cause any physiological or psychological dependence nor does it cause any adverse reaction if alcohol were to be ingested. But if you suffer from liver disease, you must notify your doctor. The drug is usually effective within an hour. It is effective for about twenty-four hours with its peak at approximately twelve hours. It should be taken at the same time every day or each time as directed. It is not recommended for prolonged use; it should not be taken for longer than a few months. It may require gradual reduction if taken longer than that. Take the drug with liquid or food to reduce potential stomach irritation. Do not drive a car or operate machinery that requires alertness and good motor coordination until the drug's effects are known. Do not take cough medications with dextromethorphan, analgesics, synthetic codeine (PERCODAN), or antidiarrheal medications (paregoric).

Pregnancy: Category C (see sidebar on page 69). While this drug enjoys a category C rating, it should not be used if the patient is or becomes pregnant unless the physician believes there is no other way the unborn child can be spared exposure to the drug of the addicted mother.

COGNITIVE ENHANCEMENT AGENT

Brand Name	Generic Name
COGNEX	tacrine (TA-kreen)

HOW THE DRUG WORKS

By increasing the levels of the neurotransmitter acetylcholine in the brain, it may reduce symptoms of Alzheimer's disease, which is thought to be caused by loss of the nerve cells that produce acetylcholine.

PURPOSE

Treatment of mild to moderate Alzheimer's disease.

DOSAGE

Treatment of Alzheimer's disease
   Adults and the Elderly: (initially) 10 mg four times daily (taken

orally), and increased every six weeks, if needed. The maximum dose is 160 mg per day.

SIDE EFFECTS

Common: Headaches; muscle aches; nausea; diarrhea; dizziness; insomnia; loss of appetite; edema of the lower limbs.

Uncommon: Facial swelling; weight gain; dehydration; confusion; increased sweating; difficulty swallowing.

ADVERSE REACTIONS

Agitation; hallucinations; excessive urination; bruises. *Rare:* slow heartbeat and abnormal heart rhythm.

DRUG INTERACTION

Increases the effects of muscle relaxants, such as succinylcholine, and bethanechol (medication for urinary-tract infections) and theophylline (anti-asthma medication).

Decreases the effects of anticholinergic medications.

TAGAMET may increase the effects of tacrine by as much as 50 percent.

OVERDOSAGE

If any of the following symptoms develop, notify your physician immediately: Intense nausea and vomiting; severe muscle weakness; slow heartbeat; hypotension; collapse; and convulsions.

Comments: Introduced in 1993, tacrine is the only drug proved to raise acetylcholine levels and to be effective in treating Alzheimer's disease. While it may take as much as a month before the drug will be effective, studies suggest that as many as 25 percent of all people who take it will be helped. Continued use of the drug often causes it to lose its effectiveness. Unfortunately, not everyone can tolerate the drug and the medication will have to be discontinued. Furthermore, the drug should not be taken if you have a history of bronchial asthma, hyperthyroidism, a urinary-tract obstruction, peptic ulcers, low blood pressure, or a slow heartbeat. Your doctor also needs to know if you have had a history of seizures or liver disease or if, during use of the drug, there is a change in your stool color, whether lighter or darker. Because women are known to experience more dose-related side effects with this drug than men, doses may be lower for them.

When preparing to discontinue its use, do not stop abruptly. This can result in confusion and cognitive dysfunction. Rather, doses should be gradually reduced over a week or more. And it is best that the drug not be taken with food.

Pregnancy: Category C (see sidebar on page 69). This means that whatever risk the drug could conceivably pose for the fetus is outweighed by the possible benefits of the drug to the mother.

HYPNOTIC SEDATIVES

Broadly speaking, hypnotics are drugs which reduce pain—such as analgesics, anesthetics, intoxicants, and sedatives. Despite the association with their name, they are not drugs that hypnotize people. The Greek word *hypnos* means *sleep.* Hence, in the context of psychiatric drugs, hypnotics refer to sedatives used to induce sleep.

The three categories of hypnotic sedatives are barbiturates, nonbarbiturates, and benzodiazepines. In their order of development: barbiturates were first introduced in the 1920s; drugs in the second group, referred to here as nonbarbiturates, were developed and used over the past thirty years; the newest group of sedatives, benzodiazepines, came on the market in the early 1970s.

Barbiturates have a wider and more powerful effect on the central nervous system than the other sedatives. They can be used to treat insomnia and, in addition, are used to calm agitated patients, to lessen anxiety prior to surgery, and to treat certain types of seizures. They have been supplanted, generally, by the newer nonbarbiturates and benzodiazepine drugs, which are more effective—while less likely to cause slower pulse or breathing rate and hangover.

Nonbarbiturates usually cause the kind of drowsiness that helps people who occasionally have difficulty in falling asleep. Primarily, they shorten the period needed to get to sleep and increase the likelihood of uninterrupted sleep. They also provide an antianxiety effect which is helpful when insomnia is accompanied by anxiety. They are usually prescribed in conjunction with nonpharmacologic treatment, such as behavioral techniques, sleep hygiene, and relaxation exercises.

Some of the nonbarbiturates promote sleep in other circumstances: PARAL is used to quiet and produce sleep in those patients suffering from delirium tremens (DTs); NOCTEC is prescribed to reduce anxiety and produce sleep in patients *before* surgery. (NOCTEC may also be used to control pain *after* surgery.)

Benzodiazepines are short-acting sedatives that produce fewer side effects than barbiturates and many of the other nonbarbiturates. Because these drugs are dependent-forming, they are prescribed only in the treatment of short-term insomnia, that is, the drug should not be used for more than two weeks. (See "Insomnia," page 49.)

Note: Although some pharmaceutical companies have established benzodiazepines as anxiolytics (antianxiety drugs) and other companies place them among hypnotics (sedatives), the distinction is arbitrary since any benzodiazepine can be used to treat either anxiety or insomnia. Hence, your doctor may use VALIUM or ATIVAN, which are benzodiazepines, at night for the treatment of insomnia even though they are listed as antianxiety agents and not hypnotic sedatives.

Course of Treatment
The effects of both these sedative medications usually occur in this manner:

1. Within a few days, the medication should help you get to sleep and stay asleep.
2. Within two weeks, however, the drug should be withdrawn. At this point, if the symptoms of the sleep disorder return, your doctor may want to explore the cause of the insomnia.

Potential Risks

All sedative drugs have some risks associated with their use, and some people are at greater risk than others.

Children Sedatives should always be used carefully with children. Some children may become irritable, excitable, tearful, or aggressive while taking barbiturates. Nonbarbiturates generally should not be given to anyone under the age of sixteen.

Women Studies have shown that barbiturates may adversely affect the fetus; they should be used only if clearly needed and the potential benefits outweigh the possible risks. On the other hand, benzodiazepines should not be used at all during a pregnancy. The one exception among these sedative drugs is NOLUDAR; studies have not shown any risk exists for the pregnant woman. However, no drug should be taken during a pregnancy unless clearly needed, and then only under a doctor's supervision. If you intend to breast-feed, consult with your doctor since (1) barbiturates, (2) benzodiazepines, and (3) one nonbarbiturate, NOCTEC, appear in breast milk. (See "Pregnant and Lactating Women," page 66.)

Elderly Because of the alterations in metabolism that occur with age, only half the normal adult recommended dose of hypnotic sedatives should be given to the elderly. Even normal doses may make some elderly patients overly sedated, dizzy, and confused. (See "The Elderly," page 72.)

Tolerance

One of the principal risks associated with these drugs is related to their continued use since, over time, your body can develop a tolerance to the drug, which means it becomes less effective. Tolerance to these drugs develops in as little as three or four weeks. When tolerance develops, some people are tempted to increase the dosage to maintain the drug's effectiveness, a practice that can lead directly to a habit-forming dependence. Consequently, do not exceed your prescribed dosage; do not use for consecutive periods of more than two weeks; and do not stop the drug abruptly.

Withdrawal

If these drugs are abruptly stopped after long-term use or high-dose therapy, you may experience the following withdrawal symptoms:

1. Within twelve hours after you have taken your last dose of a barbiturate, some minor symptoms may develop— usually in this order: anxiety, muscle twitching, tremor of hands and fingers, growing weakness, visual problems, vomiting, insomnia and orthostatic hypotension.
2. Within eighteen hours, more serious symptoms may appear, such as convulsions and delirium. Depending upon how long and how much of the barbiturates were taken, these symptoms can last as long as four or five days. Even if you taper the use of the drug, you may experience a little irritability, sleeplessness, or nervousness for a few days.

Food-and-Drug Interactions

Barbiturates may increase vitamin D and vitamin C requirements. As a measure of protection, you are advised to take 100 mg of vitamin C and 400 mg to 800 mg of vitamin D daily while taking barbiturates.

Side Effects

Physiological Effects of Hypnotic Sedatives

Behavioral Drowsiness; dizziness; confusion; strange behavior; excitement; anxiety; nervousness; insomnia; hallucinations.

Blood system Abnormal blood count.

Circulatory system (Barbiturates) slowed heart rate; hypotension. (Benzodiazepines) heart palpitations; chest pains; rapid heart rate; hypotension.

Dermatological Unusual bleeding or bruising; rash; hives; redness or yellowness.

Digestive system Nausea; vomiting, constipation; diarrhea; stomach pain; rectal gas.

Eyes Blurred vision; double vision.

Liver   Yellowing of the skin or eyes (jaundice); abnormal liver function tests.

Nervous system   Headaches; fatigue; poor coordination; poor concentration; hangovers.

Other   Unpleasant taste; unpleasant breath (PARAL); fevers; nosebleeds.

Guidelines for Use

In evaluating patients, a previous history of sedative use and abuse is important in determining the use and choice of drug.

Barbiturates   While taking these drugs, avoid alcohol use and other drugs, such as narcotic pain relievers, tranquilizers, and antihistamines. Contact your doctor if you experience symptoms such as chest pains, irregular heartbeats, blurred vision, fever, mouth sores, bruising or bleeding, yellowing of the eyes or skin. Barbiturates suppress REM sleep (*Rapid Eye Movement* or natural sleep); these drugs can cause increased dreaming or nightmares when you stop taking them. Also, use extreme caution while driving or using machinery that requires alertness or good coordination, and do not stop taking the drug abruptly.

Nonbarbiturates and benzodiazepines   Your sleep may be interrupted for a few nights following discontinuation of these drugs. Always call your doctor if the drug causes any side effects that persist for more than a week.

HYPNOTIC SEDATIVES

BARBITURATES

Brand Name	Generic Name
AMYTAL	amobarbital (am-o-BAR-bi-tal)
SECONAL	secobarbital (see-ko-BAR-bi-tal)
NEMBUTAL	pentobarbital (pen-toe-BAR-bi-tal)
AMBIEN	zolpidem (zol-PEE-dem)

NONBARBITURATES

Brand Name	Generic Name
NOCTEC	chloral hydrate (klor-al HY-drate)
NOLUDAR, AQUACHLORAL SUPPRETTES	methyprylon (meth-i-PRYE-lon)
PLACIDYL	ethchlorvynol (eth-klor-VI-nole)
DORIDEN	glutethimide (gloo-TETH-i-mide)
VALMID	ethinamate (e-THIN-a-mate)
PARAL	paraldehyde (par-AL-de-hide)

BENZODIAZEPINES

Brand Name	Generic Name
DALMANE	flurazepam (flure-AZ-e-pam)
RESTORIL, RAZEPAM	temazepam (tem-AZ-e-pam)
HALCION	triazolam (trye-AY-zoe-lam)
DORAL	quazepam (GWA-zee-pam)

BARBITURATES

Brand Name	Generic Name
AMYTAL	amobarbital (am-o-BAR-bi-tal)

HOW THE DRUG WORKS

By interfering with the production of norepinephrine, this drug probably blocks the transmission of nerve impulses from the thalamus to the cortex of the brain.

PURPOSE

Short-term insomnia (one to two weeks); sedation, prior to surgery.

DOSAGE

Treatment of insomnia

Adults: (Tablets) 100 mg to 200 mg (taken orally) with increases in dosage, if needed. (Capsules) 65 mg to 200 mg (taken orally) at bedtime.

Daytime sedation

Adults: (Tablets) 15 mg to 120 mg (taken orally) in divided doses; usual sedative dose is 30 mg to 50 mg.

SIDE EFFECTS

Common: Drowsiness; dizziness; clumsiness; hangovers.
Uncommon: Anxiety; constipation; fainting feeling; nausea; nightmares or insomnia; unusual irritability.

ADVERSE REACTIONS

Confusion; depression; unusual excitement; hallucinations; bleeding and bruising. (With long-term use): bone pain; loss of appetite; weight loss; yellowing of the eyes and skin. *Rare:* bleeding of the lips; chest pain; scaly skin; tightness in the chest; fever and mouth sores; paradoxical excitability.

DRUG INTERACTION

Increases the effects of drugs such as alcohol and other CNS depressants; narcotic analgesics; antihistamines; tranquilizers.
Decreases the effects of oral anticoagulants; cortisone drugs; oral contraceptives.

OVERDOSAGE

If any of the following symptoms develops, notify your physician immediately: Confusion; shortness of breath; trouble breathing; slurred speech; staggering; insomnia; unusual irritability; unusual eye movements; severe weakness.

Comments: Amobarbital has been an effective sedating drug since 1925; but because barbiturates are highly *addicting*, it has been largely replaced by benzodiazepines for the treatment of insomnia. Because of its dependent properties and its short-term effectiveness as a bedtime sedative (it develops a progressive tolerance with reduced effectiveness at the same dose), AMYTAL should not be used for more than two weeks. This drug is more effective in preventing interrupted sleep than at getting you to sleep. (See SECONAL, below.) Women should be advised that this drug can reduce the effectiveness of oral contraceptives.

Withdrawal from the drug should always be gradual since stopping abruptly can produce symptoms such as hallucinations, trembling, anxiety, vision problems, seizures, nightmares, and other sleeping problems. Even if you discontinue this drug by tapering its use, after a regimen of high doses for an extended period your body may need an adjustment of two weeks before you are free of any symptoms (for example, hangovers). Dreaming and nightmares are not uncommon when the drug is stopped since it suppresses REM sleep. In all cases, if you experience these or any symptoms that are troubling, call your doctor. Finally, do not exceed recommended dosages; *an overdose can be lethal.*

Pregnancy: Category B (see sidebar on page 69). This means that the risk to the fetus is relatively low.

Brand Name	*Generic Name*
SECONAL	secobarbital (see-ko-BAR-bi-tal)

HOW THE DRUG WORKS

Binds on the gaba-benzodiazepine complex—at a site apart from the benzodiazepine sedatives—to shorten sleep latency and reduce intermittent awakening.

PURPOSE

Short-term insomnia (one to two weeks); sedation, prior to surgery.

DOSAGE

Treatment of insomnia
Adults: 100 mg (taken orally) at bedtime for up to two weeks.

Sedation
Adults: 200 mg to 300 mg (taken orally), one to two hours before surgery.

Children: 2 mg to 6 mg/kg (taken orally) up to 100 mg, one to two hours before surgery.

SIDE EFFECTS

Common: Drowsiness; dizziness; clumsiness; hangovers.

Uncommon: Anxiety; constipation; fainting feeling; nausea; nightmares or insomnia; unusual irritability.

ADVERSE REACTIONS

Confusion; depression; unusual excitement; hallucinations; bleeding and bruising. (With long-term use): bone pain; loss of appetite; weight loss; yellowing of the eyes and skin. *Rare:* bleeding of the lips; chest pain; scaly skin; tightness in the chest; fever and mouth sores; paradoxical excitability.

DRUG INTERACTION

Increases the effects of drugs such as alcohol and other CNS depressants; narcotic analgesics; antihistamines; tranquilizers.

Decreases the effects of oral anticoagulants; cortisone drugs; oral contraceptives.

OVERDOSAGE

If any of the following symptoms develops, notify your physician immediately: Confusion; shortness of breath; trouble breathing; slurred speech; staggering; insomnia; unusual irritability; unusual eye movements; severe weakness.

Comments: Barbiturates like SECONAL have been around since the 1920s, but because they are highly *addicting*, they have been largely replaced by benzodiazepines for the treatment of insomnia. Because of its dependent properties and its short-term effectiveness as a bedtime sedative (it develops a progressive tolerance with reduced effectiveness at the same dose), SECONAL should not be used for more than two weeks. This drug is more effective in putting you to sleep than in preventing interrupted sleep. (See AMYTAL, page 194.) Doses of more than 400 mg for ninety days produces a physical dependence. Women should be advised that this drug can reduce the effectiveness of oral contraceptives.

Withdrawal from the drug should always be gradual. Stopping abruptly can produce symptoms such as hallucinations, trembling, anxiety, vision problems, seizures, nightmares, and other sleeping problems. Even if you discontinue this drug by tapering its use after a regimen of high doses for an extended period, your body may need an adjustment of two weeks before you are free of any symptoms (for example, hangovers). Dreaming and nightmares are not uncommon when the drug is stopped, since it suppresses REM sleep. In all cases, if you experience these or any symptoms that are troubling, call your doctor. Finally, do not exceed the recommended dosage; *an overdose can be lethal.*

Pregnancy: Category D (see sidebar on page 69). This means that studies in pregnant women have shown a significant risk to the fetus. Therefore, the drug should be used only if needed in a serious disease and when other, safer drugs have proven to be ineffective or cannot be used.

Brand Name	Generic Name
NEMBUTAL (sodium capsules and solution)	pentobarbital (pen-toe-BAR-bi-tal)

HOW THE DRUG WORKS

Binds on the gaba-benzodiazepine complex—at a site apart from the benzodiazepine sedatives—to shorten sleep latency and reduce intermittent awakening.

PURPOSE

Short-term insomnia (one to two weeks); daytime sedation.

DOSAGE

Treatment of insonᵢᵢa
  Adults: (capsules) 100 mg to 200 mg or (solution) 5 ml at bedtime for up to two weeks.

Sedation
  Adults: 20 mg to 40 mg (taken orally).

SIDE EFFECTS

Common: Drowsiness; dizziness; clumsiness; hangovers.
Uncommon: Anxiety; constipation; fainting feeling; nausea; nightmares or insomnia; unusual irritability.

ADVERSE REACTIONS

Confusion; depression; unusual excitement; hallucinations; bleeding and bruising. (With long-term use): bone pain; loss of appetite; weight loss; yellowing of the eyes and skin. *Rare:* bleeding of the lips; chest pain; scaly skin; tightness in the chest; fever and mouth sores.

DRUG INTERACTION

Increases the effects of drugs such as alcohol and other CNS depressants; narcotic analgesics; monoamine-oxidase inhibitors; antihistamines; tranquilizers.

Decreases the effects of oral anticoagulants; cortisone drugs; oral contraceptives.

OVERDOSAGE

If any of the following symptoms develops, notify your physician immediately: Confusion; shortness of breath; trouble breathing; slurred speech; staggering; insomnia; unusual irritability; unusual eye movements; severe weakness.

Comments: Barbiturates like NEMBUTAL have been around since the 1920s, but because they are highly addicting, they have been largely replaced by benzodiazepines for the treatment of insomnia. Because of its dependent properties and its short-term effectiveness as a bedtime sedative (it develops a progressive tolerance with reduced effectiveness at the same dose), NEMBUTAL should not be used for more than two weeks. Women should be advised that this drug can reduce the effectiveness of oral contraceptives.

Withdrawal from the drug should always be gradual. Stopping abruptly can produce symptoms such as hallucinations, trembling, anxiety, vision problems, seizures, nightmares, and other sleeping problems. Even if you discontinue this drug by tapering its use after a regimen of high doses for an extended period, your body may need an adjustment of two weeks before you are free of any symptoms (e.g., hangovers). Dreaming and nightmares are not uncommon when the drug is stopped, since it suppresses REM sleep. In all cases, if you experience these or any symptoms that are troubling, call your doctor. Finally, do not exceed recommended dosages; *an overdose can be lethal.*

Pregnancy: Category D (see sidebar on page 69). This means that studies in pregnant women have shown a significant risk to the fetus. Therefore, the drug should be used only if needed in a serious disease and when other, safer drugs have proven to be ineffective or cannot be used.

———————

Brand Name	*Generic Name*
AMBIEN	zolpidem (zol-PEE-dem)

HOW THE DRUG WORKS

By binding to a specific gaba-benzodiazepine receptor, it induces a hypnotic-sedative state.

PURPOSE

To induce and prolong sleep.

DOSAGE

Adults: 10 mg daily, taken before bedtime. Drug should be reevaluated after ten days' use.
Elderly: 5 mg daily.

SIDE EFFECTS

Common: Daytime drowsiness; dizziness; headache; nausea.
Uncommon: Vomiting; diarrhea; difficulty breathing; fatigue; high blood pressure; rapid heartbeat; edema.

ADVERSE REACTIONS

Skin rash; hallucinations. *Rare:* blurred vision and muscle tremors. Possibility of drug dependence and concomitant withdrawal symptoms, such as irritability and grand mal seizures.

DRUG INTERACTION

Increases effectiveness of THORAZINE, narcotics, and other CNS depressants.

Consult with your doctor before combining with TOFRANIL (imipramine).

OVERDOSAGE

If any of the following symptoms develop, notify your physician immediately: Cardiovascular and respiratory problems, impairment of consciousness from somnolence to light coma.

Comments: Introduced in 1993, the drug is used only for the treatment of insomnia. The drug should not be used beyond a ten-day period since it will gradually be less effective, which could increase the risk of dependency. It is probably advisable not to take the drug on an overnight flight since some people have experienced "traveler's amnesia." Some individuals have reported a slight memory loss with its use.
When the drug becomes ineffective, there is a risk of drug dependence in vulnerable individuals and therefore should not be used by people with a history of addiction. However, the drug is thought to

have less of an addiction liability than benzodiazepine sedative hypnotics. Notify your doctor if you have had a history of liver or kidney disease or experience any withdrawal symptoms, such as cramps or nausea. You should exercise caution when driving or operating heavy machinery when first using the drug.

Pregnancy: Category B (see sidebar on page 69). This means that the risk to the fetus is assumed to be relatively low. The effects of this drug during pregnancy, however, have not been studied. Hence, notify your doctor if you plan to become pregnant.

NONBARBITURATES

Brand Name	*Generic Name*
NOCTEC	chloral hydrate (klor-al HY-drate)

HOW THE DRUG WORKS

Not well established. Its sedative effects may be caused by acting on the sleep center of the brain.

PURPOSE

Short-term insomnia (one to two weeks).

DOSAGE

Treatment of insomnia
  Adults: 500 mg (taken orally) fifteen to thirty minutes before bedtime in divided doses following a meal.
  Children: 50 mg (taken orally) before bedtime.

Sedation
  Adults: 500 mg to 1 gram, fifteen to thirty minutes before bedtime or thirty minutes before surgery.

SIDE EFFECTS

Common: Nausea, stomach pain, vomiting, diarrhea.
Uncommon: Dizziness, unsteadiness, *hangover* in the morning.

ADVERSE REACTIONS

Skin rash or hives; confusion; hallucinations; paradoxical excitement.

DRUG INTERACTION

Increases the effects of drugs such as alcohol and other CNS depressants; narcotic analgesics.

With oral anticoagulants (*blood thinners*), this drug increases the bleeding.

OVERDOSAGE

If any of the following symptoms develops, notify your physician immediately: Excessive sleepiness; confusion; poor coordination; slurred speech; flushed skin; coma.

Comments: Introduced in 1860, NOCTEC is one of the oldest therapeutic drugs still on the market. Over the years it has enjoyed various street names, such as a *Mickey* or *Peter* and, when combined with alcohol, *knockout drops* and *Mickey Finn*. It is an *addicting* drug, but when used correctly, it remains a highly respectable sedative.

As a liquid, the drug can be taken with fruit juice to reduce its unpleasant taste and reduce the risk of stomach irritation. If you take capsules do not chew them: swallow them whole.

Avoid alcohol while taking this drug; it could increase sedation. Avoid drinking more than one cup of coffee or tea per day (and never at night); the caffeine can reduce the sleep-inducing effect of the drug. Do not smoke (especially at night) since nicotine is a stimulant that may reduce the drug's effectiveness.

Pregnancy: Category C (see sidebar on page 69). This means that whatever risk the drug could conceivably pose for the fetus is outweighed by the possible benefits of the drug to the mother. However, you are advised to avoid its use during the first trimester of a pregnancy, whenever possible.

Brand Name	*Generic Name*
NOLUDAR,	methyprylon (meth-
AQUACHLORAL	i-PRYE-lon)
SUPPRETTES	

HOW THE DRUG WORKS

By raising the threshold of the arousal centers in the brain, this drug causes sedation.

PURPOSE

Short-term insomnia (one to two weeks).

DOSAGE

Treatment of insomnia

   Adults: 200 mg to 400 mg (taken orally) fifteen minutes before bedtime.

   Children under twelve years: initially, 50 mg (taken orally) before bedtime; if necessary, it can be increased up to 200 mg at bedtime.

SIDE EFFECTS

   Common: Drowsiness; dizziness; headaches.
   Uncommon: Diarrhea; nausea; vomiting.

ADVERSE REACTIONS

Skin rash or hives; confusion; hallucinations; trembling.

DRUG INTERACTION

Increases the effects of drugs such as alcohol and other CNS depressants; narcotic analgesics.

OVERDOSAGE

   If any of the following symptoms develops, notify your physician immediately: Confusion, poor balance or staggering walk; shortness of breath or difficulty breathing; excessive sleepiness; coma.

   Comments: NOLUDAR is a highly *addicting* drug that should not be used long-term if avoidable. Because it has unusual and complex metabolic routes and is fat-soluble (the drug is stored in the fat of your body), it tends to leave the body slowly; therefore, do not exceed recommended dosages, as an overdose can be lethal. As this drug suppress REM sleep (as do barbiturates), it causes increased dreaming or nightmares when it is stopped. Withdrawal from the drug should always be gradual since stopping abruptly can be dangerous.

Avoid alcohol while taking this drug; it could increase sedation. On the other hand, avoid drinking more than one cup of coffee or tea per day (and never at night); the caffeine can reduce the sleep-inducing effect of the drug. Do not smoke (especially at night) since nicotine is a stimulant that may reduce the drug's effectiveness.

Pregnancy: Category B (see sidebar on page 69). This means that the risk to the fetus is relatively low.

Brand Name	*Generic Name*
PLACIDYL	ethchlorvynol (eth-klor-VI-nole)

HOW THE DRUG WORKS

Not well understood, but it is thought to act in the wake-sleep centers of the brain.

PURPOSE

Short-term insomnia (one to two weeks).

DOSAGE

Treatment of insomnia
   Adults: (depending upon severity of insomnia) 500 mg (taken orally) before bedtime, up to a week; for patients who are switching from another hypnotic, 750 mg at bedtime; (for severe insomnia) 1,000 mg (1 gram) at bedtime.

SIDE EFFECTS

Common: Blurred vision; dizziness; indigestion, nausea; fatigue.
Uncommon: Confusion; daytime drowsiness; unsteadiness.

ADVERSE REACTIONS

Skin rash or hives; bleeding or bruising; nervousness or restlessness. *Rare:* yellowing of the skin or eyes, itching, and dark urine (indications of drug-induced hepatitis).

DRUG INTERACTION

Increases the effects of drugs such as alcohol and other CNS depressants; narcotic analgesics; tricyclic antidepressants; monoamine-oxidase (MAO) inhibitors.

With oral anticoagulants, it may increase the thinning of the blood.

OVERDOSAGE

If any of the following symptoms develops, notify your physician immediately: Confusion; poor balance or staggering walk; shortness of breath or difficulty breathing; double vision; trembling; slurred speech; unusually slow heartbeat.

Comments: PLACIDYL is a highly addicting drug that may not be effective if used for much more than seven consecutive days. Because this drug has unusual and complex metabolic routes and is fat-soluble (the drug is stored in the fat of your body), it tends to exit the body slowly. Do not exceed the recommended dosage; an overdose can be lethal. Withdrawal from the drug should be gradual since stopping abruptly can be dangerous.

This drug has an unpleasant aftertaste, but milk or food will mask the unpleasant taste and reduce the potential giddiness and stomach upset it causes (since the food slows the drug's rapid absorption).

Avoid alcohol while taking this drug; it could increase sedation. On the other hand, avoid drinking more than one cup of coffee or tea per day (and never at night); the caffeine can reduce the sleep-inducing effect of the drug. Do not smoke (especially at night) since nicotine is a stimulant that may reduce the drug's effectiveness.

Pregnancy: Category C (see sidebar on page 69). This means that whatever risk the drug could conceivably pose for the fetus is outweighed by the possible benefits of the drug to the mother. However,

you are advised to avoid its use during the first trimester of a pregnancy, whenever possible. _____

Brand Name	Generic Name
DORIDEN	glutethimide (gloo-TETH-i-mide)

HOW THE DRUG WORKS

Not well understood, but thought to act in the wake-sleep centers of the brain.

PURPOSE

Short-term insomnia (one to two weeks).

DOSAGE

Treatment of insomnia
   Adults: 0.25 gram to 0.5 gram (taken orally) before bedtime, up to a week.

SIDE EFFECTS

   Common: (daytime) Drowsiness.
   Uncommon: Blurred vision; confusion; dizziness; hangovers; nausea.

ADVERSE REACTIONS

Skin rash. *Rare:* bleeding or bruising; nervousness or unusual excitability; excessive fatigue; sore throat and fever.

DRUG INTERACTION

Increases the effects of drugs such as alcohol and other CNS depressants; narcotic analgesics.

With oral anticoagulants, it may increase the thinning of the blood.

OVERDOSAGE

   If any of the following symptoms develops, notify your physician immediately: Bluish color to the skin; persistent confusion; fevers.

Comments: DORIDEN is a highly addicting drug that is not effective if used for much more than seven consecutive days. Because it has unusual and complex metabolic routes and is fat-soluble (the drug is stored in the fat of your body), it tends to exit the body slowly. Do not exceed the recommended dosage; an overdose can be lethal. As this drug suppresses REM sleep (as do barbiturates), it causes increased dreaming or nightmares when it is stopped. Withdrawal from the drug should always be gradual since stopping abruptly can be dangerous. Call your doctor if a rash develops: you may have an allergic reaction.

Avoid alcohol while taking this drug; it could increase sedation. Avoid drinking more than one cup of coffee or tea per day (and never at night); the caffeine can reduce the sleep-inducing effect of the drug. Do not smoke (especially at night) since nicotine is a stimulant that may reduce the drug's effectiveness.

Pregnancy: Category C (see sidebar on page 69). This means that whatever risk the drug could conceivably pose for the fetus is outweighed by the possible benefits of the drug to the mother. However, you are advised to avoid its use during the first trimester of a pregnancy, whenever possible.

Brand Name	*Generic Name*
VALMID	ethinamate (e-THIN-a-mate)

HOW THE DRUG WORKS

Not well understood, but it is thought to act in the wake-sleep centers of the brain.

PURPOSE

Short-term insomnia (one to two weeks).

DOSAGE

Treatment of insomnia

Adults: 500 mg to 1,000 mg (taken orally) twenty minutes before bedtime, up to a week.

Elderly: initially, 250 mg (same initial dose for debilitated patients).

Note: To diminish the dose, the 500-mg capsule can be cut in half, emptied in water, and drunk.

SIDE EFFECTS

Common: None.
Uncommon: Upset stomach; nausea.

ADVERSE REACTIONS

Skin rash; unusual excitability. *Rare:* bleeding or bruising.

DRUG INTERACTION

Increases the effects of drugs such as alcohol and other CNS depressants.

OVERDOSAGE

If any of the following symptoms develops, notify your physician immediately: Confusion; shortness of breath; trouble breathing; slurred speech; staggering; slow heartbeat; severe weakness.

Comments: VALMID is a highly addicting drug that is not effective if used for much more than seven consecutive days. Because this drug has unusual and complex metabolic routes, and is fat-soluble (the drug is stored in the fat of your body), it tends to exit the body slowly. Therefore, do not exceed recommended dosages; *an overdose can be lethal.* Withdrawal from the drug should always be gradual since stopping abruptly can produce symptoms such as hallucinations, trembling, and seizures.

Avoid alcohol while taking this drug; it could increase sedation. Avoid drinking more than one cup of coffee or tea per day (and never at night); the caffeine can reduce the sleep-inducing effect of the drug. Do not smoke (especially at night) since nicotine is a stimulant that may reduce the drug's effectiveness.

Pregnancy: Category C (see sidebar on page 69). This means that whatever risk the drug could conceivably pose for the fetus is outweighed by the possible benefits of the drug to the mother. However, you are advised to avoid its use during the first trimester of a pregnancy, whenever possible.

———————

Brand Name	*Generic Name*
PARAL	paraldehyde (par-AL-de-hide) (liquid)

HOW THE DRUG WORKS

Not well understood, but it is thought to act in the wake-sleep centers of the brain.

PURPOSE

Calm and induce sleep in patients who are nervous and tense; reduce delirium tremens (DTs) in the treatment of alcoholism withdrawal; seizures of the grand mal type.

DOSAGE

Treatment of insomnia
   Adults: (in liquid form) 10 ml to 30 ml (taken orally or rectally); 10 ml (intramuscular injection).
   Children: 0.3 ml (taken orally, rectally, or by intramuscular injection).

Sedation
   Adults: 4 ml to 10 ml (taken orally or rectally); 5 ml (intramuscular injection).
   Children: 0.15 ml (taken orally, rectally, or by intramuscular injection).

Treatment of alcohol withdrawal
   Adults: 5 ml to 10 ml (taken orally or rectally); 5 ml (intramuscular injection) every four to six hours for the first twenty-four hours, then every six hours on following days, not to exceed 40 ml (orally) or 20 ml (intramuscular injections) per twenty-four hours.

SIDE EFFECTS

Common: Drowsiness; nausea; stomach pain; bad breath.
Uncommon: Clumsiness; dizziness; hangovers.

ADVERSE REACTIONS

Skin rash. *With long-term care:* yellowing of the eyes or skin.

DRUG INTERACTION

Increases the effects of drugs such as alcohol and other CNS depressants; ANTABUSE.

OVERDOSAGE

If any of the following symptoms develops, notify your physician immediately: Confusion; decreased urination; tremors; shortness of breath; trouble breathing; hyperventilation; severe stomach cramps; slow heartbeat; severe weakness.

Comments: PARAL is a highly addicting drug that is available in liquid form. Withdrawal from the drug should always be gradual since stopping abruptly can produce symptoms such as hallucinations, trembling, seizures, and unusual sweating. This drug has a characteristic foul smell and the bad breath it causes will last until about one day after you stop using it. The oral dose should be diluted with cold fruit juice or milk to mask its taste and reduce the possibility of stomach distress.

Pregnancy: Category C (see sidebar on page 69). This means that whatever risk the drug could conceivably pose for the fetus is outweighed by the possible benefits of the drug to the mother. However, you are advised to avoid its use during the first trimester of a pregnancy, whenever possible.

BENZODIAZEPINES

Brand Name	*Generic Name*
DALMANE	flurazepam (flure-AZ-e-pam)

HOW THE DRUG WORKS

By acting on the thalamus and hypothalamus and limbic system of the brain, this drug induces sleep.

PURPOSE

Short-term insomnia (one to two weeks).

DOSAGE

Treatment of insomnia
   Adults: 15 mg to 30 mg (taken orally) before bedtime.
   Elderly: initially, 15 mg at bedtime until the patient's response is established.

SIDE EFFECTS

   Common: Dizziness; drowsiness; light-headedness; unsteadiness.
   Uncommon: diarrhea; stomachache; constipation; nausea; watery mouth; slurred speech.

ADVERSE REACTIONS

Skin rash or itching; headaches; unusual tiredness or weakness; confusion.

DRUG INTERACTION

Increases the effects of drugs such as alcohol and other CNS depressants; narcotic analgesics.

With cimetidine, it increases sedation of this drug.

OVERDOSAGE

   If any of the following symptoms develops, notify your physician immediately: Excessive sleepiness; lethargy; confusion; coma.

   Comments: DALMANE has a long half-life, which means it remains in the body longer than so-called short-acting drugs. It is metabolized in the liver into a long-acting form. (See "Active Metabolites" in the Glossary, page 287.) Its long half-life accounts both for (1) its being more effective on the third or fourth night, and (2) your *hangover* on the third or fourth morning. If the hangover continues, or daytime dizziness occurs, call your doctor. Because the *hangover* effects can impair mental alertness, use extreme caution while driving or using machinery that requires alertness or good coordination.

The length of time this drug stays in the body increases with age; hence, because of their slowed metabolism, the elderly may experience daytime sleepiness. Do not give this drug to children under the age of fifteen who are having trouble sleeping.

Avoid alcohol while taking this drug as it could increase sedation. Also avoid drinking more than one cup of coffee or tea per day (and never at night), as the caffeine can reduce the sleep-inducing effect of the drug. Do not smoke (especially at night) since nicotine is a stimulant that may reduce the drug's effectiveness.

Pregnancy: Category D (see sidebar on page 69). This means that studies in pregnant women have shown a significant risk to the fetus. Therefore, the drug should be used only if needed in a serious disease and when other, safer drugs have proven to be ineffective or cannot be used.

Brand Name	*Generic Name*
RESTORIL, RAZEPAM	temazepam (tem-AZ- e-pam)

HOW THE DRUG WORKS

By acting on the thalamus and hypothalamus and limbic system of the brain, this drug induces sleep.

PURPOSE

Short-term insomnia (one to two weeks).

DOSAGE

Treatment of insomnia
   Adults: 15 mg to 30 mg (taken orally) before bedtime.
   Elderly: initially, 15 mg at bedtime until patient's response is established.

SIDE EFFECTS

Common: Dizziness, drowsiness; light-headedness; unsteadiness.
Uncommon: Diarrhea; stomachache; constipation; nausea; watery mouth; slurred speech.

ADVERSE REACTIONS

Skin rash or itching; headaches; trouble sleeping; unusual tiredness or weakness; confusion.

DRUG INTERACTION

Increases the effects of drugs such as alcohol and other CNS depressants; narcotic analgesics.

OVERDOSAGE

If any of the following symptoms develops, notify your physician immediately: Excessive sleepiness; confusion; diminished reflexes; difficulty breathing; coma.

Comments: Since RESTORIL is absorbed slowly into the body, it must be taken thirty to sixty minutes before sleep. Some people may experience trouble sleeping the first or second night after discontinuing the medication. It should be used with great caution in individuals with liver disease.

Avoid alcohol while using this drug; it could increase sedation. Use extreme caution while driving or using machinery that requires alertness or good coordination. Also avoid drinking more than one cup of coffee or tea per day (and never at night), as the caffeine can reduce the sleep-inducing effect of the drug. Do not smoke (especially at night) since nicotine is a stimulant that may reduce the drug's effectiveness.

Pregnancy: Category X (see sidebar on page 69). This means that the drug poses such a great risk for the fetus that it should not be given (*contraindicated*) to pregnant women.

Brand Name	Generic Name
HALCION	triazolam (trye-AY-zoe-lam)

HOW THE DRUG WORKS

By acting on the thalamus, hypothalamus, and limbic system of the brain, this drug induces sleep.

PURPOSE

Short-term insomnia (one to two weeks).

DOSAGE

Treatment of insomnia

Adults: 0.125 mg to 0.25 mg (taken orally) before bedtime. The dose may be increased to 0.5 mg. (Be cautious; the likelihood of adverse reactions increases with increased dosages.)

Elderly: initially, 0.125 mg at bedtime until patient's response is established.

SIDE EFFECTS

Common: Dizziness; drowsiness; light-headedness; unsteadiness.
Uncommon: Diarrhea; stomachache; constipation; nausea; watery mouth; slurred speech.

ADVERSE REACTIONS

Skin rash or itching; menstrual irregularities; trouble sleeping; hallucinations; aggressiveness; unusual tiredness or weakness; confusion.

DRUG INTERACTION

Increases the effects of drugs such as alcohol and other CNS depressants; narcotic analgesics.

With cimetidine and erythromycin, it increases or prolongs the sedation of this drug.

With nonsedating antihistamines (e.g., SELDANE and HISMANAL), can cause a slow heartbeat.

OVERDOSAGE

If any of the following symptoms develops, notify your physician immediately: Excessive sleepiness; confusion; poor coordination; slurred speech; coma.

Comments: HALCION is a short-acting drug, that is, it works quickly and has less tendency to produce morning drowsiness. However, it can accumulate (or be stored) in some patients, particularly those with cerebral arteriosclerosis. In these instances, its sedation will increase with continued use. It is always advised to stay within the prescribed doses because adverse reactions are directly influenced by the size of the dose of this drug.

You may have trouble getting to sleep one or two nights after stopping the use of HALCION. (See "Rebound Insomnia," page 51.) It also has been known to cause withdrawal symptoms: for example, hyperexcitability, daytime anxiety, confusion, amnesia, mood disorders, and anterograde amnesia (i.e., an inability to recall things learned two to three hours after taking the drug). This drug also requires a washout period of three to five days before you can start taking another psychiatric drug.

Avoid alcohol while using this drug; it could increase sedation. Use extreme caution while driving or using machinery that requires alertness or good coordination. Also avoid drinking more than one cup of coffee or tea per day (and never at night), as the caffeine can reduce the sleep-inducing effect of the drug. Do not smoke (especially at night) since nicotine is a stimulant that may reduce the drug's effectiveness.

Some controversy surrounds the use of this drug. The press has reported complaints from users that the drug has caused amnesia, anxiety, and paranoia. In Europe, the issue surrounding the use of HALCION has been publicly debated for ten years; and France and the Netherlands have suspended the licensed sale of the drug until further clinical studies are conducted. If you have any concerns about its potential for adverse reactions, especially the possibility of sleeplessness and anxiety, share them with your doctor. If you still feel apprehensive after your conversation, ask the doctor to prescribe another drug.

Pregnancy: Category X (see sidebar on page 69). This means the drug poses such a high risk for the fetus that it is not given (is *contraindicated*) to pregnant women.

Brand Name	Generic Name
DORAL	quazepam (GWA-zee-pam)

HOW THE DRUG WORKS

By acting on the thalamus, hypothalamus, and limbic system of the brain, this drug induces sleep.

PURPOSE

Calm and induce sleep in patients who are nervous and tense; reduce delirium tremens (DTs) in the treatment of alcoholism withdrawal and other convulsive conditions, such as grand mal seizures.

DOSAGE

Treatment of insomnia
   Adults: (in liquid form) 10 ml to 30 ml (taken orally or rectally); 10 ml (intramuscular injection).
   Children: 0.3 ml (taken orally, rectally, or intramuscularly).

Sedation
   Adults: 4 ml to 10 ml (taken orally or rectally); 5 ml (intramuscular injection).
   Children: 0.15 ml (taken orally, rectally, or intramuscularly).

Treatment of alcohol withdrawal
   Adults: 5 ml to 10 ml (taken orally or rectally); 5 ml (intramuscular injection) every four to six hours for the first twenty-four hours, then every six hours on following days, not to exceed 40 ml (orally) or 20 ml (intramuscular injections) per twenty-four hours.

SIDE EFFECTS

Common: Drowsiness; nausea; stomach pain; bad breath.
Uncommon: Clumsiness; dizziness; hangovers.

ADVERSE REACTIONS

Skin rash. *With long-term care:* yellowing of the eyes or skin.

DRUG INTERACTION

Increases the effects of drugs such as alcohol and other CNS depressants; ANTABUSE.

OVERDOSAGE

If any of the following symptoms develops, notify your physician immediately: Confusion; decreased urination; tremors; shortness of breath; trouble breathing; hyperventilation; severe stomach cramps; slow heartbeat; severe weakness.

Comments: DORAL apparently does not produce many of the side effects of other benzodiazepines with long half-lives, especially the highly popular HALCION. For example, you should have little or no difficulty getting to sleep after stopping therapy. It is also less likely to cause withdrawal symptoms, such as hyperexcitability, daytime anxiety, confusion, amnesia, mood disorders, and anterograde amnesia (i.e., an inability to recall things learned two to three hours after taking the drug). However, it requires a washout period of as much as a week before you can start taking another psychiatric drug; in the elderly it may be as long as ten days. Unlike HALCION, long-term use of this drug may cause increased sedation and possibly anxiety.

Of course, avoid alcohol while using this drug; it could increase sedation. Use extreme caution while driving or using machinery that requires alertness or good coordination. Also avoid drinking more than one cup of coffee or tea per day (and never at night), as the caffeine can reduce the sleep-inducing effect of the drug. Do not

SHORT- AND LONG-ACTING
BENZODIAZEPINE HYPNOTIC DRUGS

Comparative effects of those drugs that remain in the body for a brief period (short-acting) and those that remain in the body for a longer period of time (long-acting)

Effect	Short-Acting	Long-Acting
Accumulation with repeated use	No	Marked
Daytime anxiety	Mild	None
Early-morning insomnia	Mild	None
Hangover effects the next day	Mild	Moderate
Rebound insomnia	Moderate	None
Tolerance	Moderate	Mild

smoke (especially at night) since nicotine is a stimulant that may reduce the drug's effectiveness.

Pregnancy: Category not established. Therefore, consult your doctor before using this drug.

ANTIHISTAMINES

Antihistamines were introduced in the 1940s to reduce the effects of the chemical *histamine*, secreted by hypersensitive cell tissues as part of an allergic reaction. It is thought that the drug blocks the access of the histamine to cells that would be affected, rather than blocking its secretion from the cell. The fact that these antihistamine drugs are biochemically related to the organic compound phenothiazine (found in major tranquilizers such as THORAZINE) might also account for their sedating effect (an annoying side effect for many people who used these drugs only to treat their allergies).

The sedating quality of some antihistamines makes them effective in the treatment of short-term insomnia. BENADRYL, which may appear under many other brand names or in combination with other drugs, is used to control nervous and emotional symptoms of anxiety, and both BENADRYL and PHENERGAN are used for nighttime sedation or short-term insomnia (one to two weeks). As sedatives, these drugs are considered safe and often effective. A measure of our confidence in their safety, some antihistamines are used in drop form for infants and teething babies; they are also used to treat adults for motion sickness, and short-term anxiety or apprehension associated with insomnia.

Course of Treatment

These drugs come in the form of pills, injections, and drops. They are most effective when taken thirty minutes before bedtime and are usually effective for at least seven to ten days. Beyond two weeks they begin to lose their effectiveness. Furthermore, by that time their anticholinergic properties (such as dry mouth, increased sweating, and possible urinary retention) also make them less agreeable.

Potential Risks

All drugs, including antihistamines, have some risks associated with their use, and some people are at greater risk than others.

Children Antihistamine use in children may decrease mental alertness. In the very young child, a quite opposite reaction may develop: hyperactivity. An overdose may produce hallucinations and convulsions. As a rule, therefore, never give a child under the age of twelve a prescription antihistamine without a doctor's supervision and carefully read the label of any nonprescription antihistamines for those same children.

Women Although studies have not shown that antihistamines pose a threat to the fetus, no drug should be used during pregnancy unless clearly needed. Do not breast-feed because antihistamines appear in breast milk. (See "Pregnant and Lactating Women," page 66.)

Elderly   These antihistamines are more likely to cause drowsiness, dizziness, confusion, and low blood pressure among the elderly; therefore, lower doses should be used, if possible. (See "The Elderly," page 72.)

Side Effects
The frequency and severity of side effects depend on factors such as the strength of the dose, how long someone has taken the drug, and, of course, the susceptibility of the user. (See "People at Particular Risk," page 66.) However, most antihistamine users experience few, if any, side effects—with the exception of dry mouth and throat.

Physiological Effects of Antihistamines
Behavioral   Drowsiness; dizziness; mental confusion; insomnia.

Circulatory system   Hypotension; heart palpitations; irregular heartbeat.

Dermatological   Rash; hives; excessive sweating.

Digestive system   Nausea; vomiting; constipation; diarrhea; stomachache.

Eyes and ears   Sensitivity to light; blurred vision; double vision; ringing in the ears.

Nervous system   Headaches; fatigue; poor coordination; poor concentration.

Urinary system   Difficult urination; urine retention.

Other   Sore throat; dry mouth; chills.

Guidelines for Use
When using these medications be careful if you are driving a car or using machinery that requires alertness or good coordination.

Common side effects are gastrointestinal distress and dry mouth. Take the medication with food to avoid an upset stomach; sugarless hard candy should relieve the dryness.

If PHENERGAN causes any muscle twitching or an unusual

sensitivity to the sunlight, notify your doctor. Always call your doctor if the drug causes any side effects that persist for more than a week.

ANTIHISTAMINES

Brand Name	Generic Name
BENADRYL	diphenhydramine (dee-fen-HYE-dra-meen)
PHENERGAN	promethazine (pro-METH-a-zeen)
ATARAX, ANXAMIL, ATOZINE, DURRAX, E-VISTA, HYDROXACEN, HYZINE, QUIESS, VISTACON, VISTAJET, VISTAQUEL, VISTARIL, VISTAZINE	hydroxyzine (hy-DROX-i-zeen)

ANTIHISTAMINES

Brand Name	Generic Name
BENADRYL	diphenhydramine (dee-fen-HYE-dra-meen)

HOW THE DRUG WORKS

By blocking the action of histamine, this drug prevents allergic responses (but does not reverse histamine response, especially its effects on bronchial tubes).

PURPOSE

Allergy symptoms; motion sickness; sedation (for antianxiety and parkinsonism); short-term insomnia (one to two weeks).

222

DOSAGE

Treatment of insomnia
   Adults: (taken orally) 50 mg or 20 ml (4 tsp) before bedtime.

Sedation
   Adults, including the Elderly: 25 mg to 50 mg; 10 ml to 20 ml (2 tsp to 4 tsp).

SIDE EFFECTS

   Common: Drowsiness (especially among the elderly).
   Uncommon: Blurred vision; confusion; urine retention; dizziness; dryness of the mouth; sensitivity of the skin to the sun; ringing in the ears; excessive sweating.

ADVERSE REACTIONS

Sore throat; fever; bleeding and bruising; headaches; heart palpitations; restlessness; tightness in the chest; flushing redness in face; hallucinations; insomnia; seizures.

DRUG INTERACTION

Increases the effects of drugs such as alcohol and other CNS depressants.

OVERDOSAGE

   If any of the following symptoms develops, notify your physician immediately: Excessive sleepiness; lethargy; confusion; insomnia; tremors; coma.

   Comments: Diphenhydramine has been around since 1945 as an effective medication in the treatment of allergic reactions. Because it is one of the more sedating antihistamines, it is also a popular medication in the treatment of insomnia, and the nervousness associated with anxiety.
   Avoid alcohol while taking this drug; it could increase sedation. Take it with milk or food to avoid stomach upset. On the other hand, avoid drinking more than one cup of coffee or tea per day

(and never at night); the caffeine can reduce the sleep-inducing effect of the drug. Do not smoke (especially at night), since nicotine is a stimulant that may reduce the drug's effectiveness. Sugarless gum or ice chips may relieve the symptom of dry mouth.

Pregnancy: Category C (see sidebar on page 69). This means that whatever risk the drug could conceivably pose for the fetus is outweighed by the possible benefits of the drug to the mother. However, you are advised to avoid its use during the first trimester of a pregnancy, whenever possible.

Brand Name	*Generic Name*
PHENERGAN	promethazine (pro-METH-a-zeen)

HOW THE DRUG WORKS

By blocking the action of histamine, this drug prevents allergic response (but does not reverse histamine response).

PURPOSE

Allergy symptoms; motion sickness; nausea and vomiting; nighttime sedation.

DOSAGE

Sedation
Adults: (nighttime sedation) 25 mg to 50 mg given at bedtime; (before surgery) 50 mg.
Children: (nighttime sedation) 12.5 mg to 25 mg given at bedtime.

SIDE EFFECTS

Common: Drowsiness; skin sensitive to the sun.
Uncommon: Blurred vision; decreased mental alertness (especially in children); confusion; feeling faint; dry mouth; nausea; urine retention; ringing in ears; excessive sweating.

ADVERSE REACTIONS

Sore throat; fever; bleeding and bruising; headaches; heart palpitations; restlessness; tightness in the chest; flushing redness in face; hallucinations; insomnia; seizures.

DRUG INTERACTION

Increases the effects of drugs such as alcohol and other CNS depressants.

With phenothiazine (e.g., THORAZINE), it increases sedation.

OVERDOSAGE

If any of the following symptoms develops, notify your physician immediately: Trouble breathing; excessive dizziness; coma.

Comments: As with diphenhydramine, promethazine has been around since 1945. In addition to its use as a medication for nighttime sedation, it is also effective for preoperative medication and motion sickness (car sickness).

Avoid alcohol while taking this drug; it could increase sedation. Take it with milk or food to avoid stomach upset. Also avoid drinking more than one cup of coffee or tea per day (and never at night); the caffeine can reduce the sleep-inducing effect of the drug. Do not smoke (especially at night), since nicotine is a stimulant that may reduce the drug's effectiveness. Sugarless gum or ice chips may relieve the symptom of dry mouth.

This drug should be used with great caution in children with a history of apnea (temporary stopping of breathing during sleep), a family history of sudden infant death syndrome (SIDS), or with Reye's syndrome. Do not give this drug to children under the age of two. *Never give prescription antihistamines to children under twelve unless advised by a doctor.*

Pregnancy: Category C (see sidebar on page 69). This means that whatever risk the drug could conceivably pose for the fetus is outweighed by the possible benefits of the drug to the mother. However, you are advised to avoid its use during the first trimester of a pregnancy, whenever possible. (One of its adverse reactions is a false-positive result on a pregnancy test.)

Brand Name	Generic Name
ATARAX, ANXAMIL, ATOZINE, DURRAX, E-VISTA, HYDROXACEN, HYZINE, QUIESS, VISTACON, VISTAJET, VISTAQUEL, VISTARIL, VISTAZINE	hydroxyzine (hy-DROX-i-zeen)

HOW THE DRUG WORKS

By blocking the action of histamine and depressing the CNS at certain areas (limbic) of the brain, this drug reduces anxiety.

PURPOSE

Anxiety and tension associated with psychoneurosis; anxiety associated with organic disease; preoperative sedation; commonly used by dermatologists for a variety of conditions, including itching (used as an antipruritic).

DOSAGE

Treatment of anxiety and tension
  Adults: (taken orally) 50 mg to 100 mg daily in divided doses.
  Children over six years: 50 mg to 100 mg daily in divided doses.
  Children under six years: 50 mg daily in divided doses.

SIDE EFFECTS

Common: Drowsiness (especially among the elderly).
Uncommon: Dry mouth.

ADVERSE REACTIONS

Rare: Seizures; skin rash; trembling or shakiness.

DRUG INTERACTION

Increases the effects of drugs such as alcohol and other CNS depressants.

OVERDOSAGE

If any of the following symptoms develops, notify your physician immediately: Excessive sleepiness; hypotension.

Comments: Because of its sedating side effect, hydroxyzine is used in the treatment of anxiety and tension. It is also used to treat allergic itching that may cause insomnia.

Avoid alcohol while taking this drug; it could increase sedation. Drinking more than one cup of coffee or tea per day may reduce the sedating effect of the drug. While taking this drug, it is advised that you do not drive a car or operate machinery that requires alertness or good coordination unless necessary. Sugarless gum or ice chips may relieve the symptom of dry mouth.

Pregnancy: Category C (see sidebar on page 69). This means that whatever risk the drug could conceivably pose for the fetus is outweighed by the possible benefits of the drug to the mother. However, you are advised to avoid its use during the first trimester of a pregnancy, whenever possible.

ANTIDYSKINETICS

Antidyskinetics are drugs that have been borrowed from the field of neurology and are used especially for the treatment of the movement disorders associated with the disease of parkinsonism. Some antidyskinetic drugs have actually been prescribed since the 19th century, although without any scientific rationale, other than they seemed to relieve symptoms of abnormal movements. Of the drugs discussed here COGENTIN has been used since the 1950s, while ARTANE and SYMMETREL only recently have been introduced.

The symptoms of abnormal movement occur when an imbalance between the dopamine and cholinergic nervous systems develops. For example, if a drug blocks one system, such as the major antipsychotic dopamine blocker HALDOL, it will increase the influence of the cholinergic system. The resulting imbalance could potentially produce symptoms of abnormal movements or what are called extrapyramidal symptoms. ARTANE and COGENTIN address this problem by blocking the cholinergic output. In other circumstances SYMMETREL, which increases the dopamine output, would be the drug of choice. SYMMETREL is also an antiviral agent.

Course of Treatment

The goal of antidyskinetic drugs is to control drug-induced parkinsonian symptoms that result from the use of another psychiatric drug.

With adults taking major tranquilizers, these antidyskinetic drugs are introduced only when extrapyramidal symptoms appear. In practice, this means that the drugs are usually not required for at least a week or two after tranquilizer use begins. Antidyskinetic drugs are frequently not needed after one or two months of major tranquilizer use, since patients generally develop a tolerance to the muscle stiffness. However, as many as 25% of all people using major tranquilizers may require long-term use of antidyskinetic drugs.

If major tranquilizers are used by children or adolescents, the antidyskinetic drugs are given simultaneously with the major tranquilizer because these people are at especially high risk of damage caused by extrapyramidal symptoms.

Potential Risks

The use of antidyskinetic drugs pose potential risks for everyone, but some people are at greater risk than others.

Children   COGENTIN should not be used in children under the age of three. The safety and effectiveness for children under the age of twelve have not been established.

Women   The safety of all these drugs for use during pregnancy has not been established. It is recommended that they be used only if clearly needed and potential benefits outweigh the possible hazards. Speak to your physician about its use during pregnancy. Also, if you intend to breast-feed, consult your doctor; these drugs are known to appear in breast milk. (See "Pregnant and Lactating Women," page 66.)

Elderly People over the age of sixty are more susceptible to a variety of side effects, especially mental confusion, disorientation, agitation, and hallucination.

Food and Drug Interactions
The use of COGENTIN could conceivably cause constipation. Hence, after first consulting with your physician, it may be helpful to increase both the amount of fluid you usually drink and the bulk in your diet. Avoid the use of alcohol while taking these drugs.

Side Effects
The frequency and severity of side effects or adverse reactions depend on factors such as the strength of the dose, how long someone has taken the drug and, of course, the susceptibility of the user (see "People at Particular Risk," page 66).

Physiological Effects of Antidyskinetics
Behavioral Disorientation; confusion; memory loss; hallucinations; nervousness; excitement; depression; sleeplessness.

Circulatory system Rapid heart rate; pounding in chest; low blood pressure; irregular heartbeat; light-headedness or dizziness.

Dermatological Flushing; rash; both an increase or decrease in sweating; hives.

Digestive system Nausea; vomiting; diarrhea; gas; loss of appetite; constipation; diarrhea.

Eyes Blurred vision; double vision; glaucoma.

Muscular system Twitching movement of face, eyelids, mouth, hands or legs; hand tremor.

Guidelines for Use
Always call your doctor if the drug causes any side effects that persist for more than a week. Do not hesitate to notify your doctor

if you experience involuntary muscle twitching, signs of jaundice (e.g., yellowing of the eyes and skin), skin rash, impaired vision, or irregular heartbeats.

ANTIDYSKINETICS

Brand Name	*Generic Name*
ARTANE, TRIHEXANE, TRIHEXY	trihexyphenidyl (try-hex-e-FEN-i-dill)
SYMMETREL	amantadine (a-MAN-ta-deen)
COGENTIN	benztropine (BENZ-tro-peen)

ANTIDYSKINETICS

Brand Name	*Generic Name*
ARTANE, TRIHEXANE, TRIHEXY	trihexyphenidyl (try-hex-e-FEN-i-dill)

HOW THE DRUG WORKS

By blocking the central cholinergic receptors, this drug helps to control the chemical imbalance that causes the symptoms of parkinsonism.

PURPOSE

Parkinsonism; drug-induced extrapyramidal disturbances.

DOSAGE

Treatment of parkinsonism

Adults: (initially) 1 mg (taken orally) daily, followed by, if needed, increases of 2 mg daily in three- to five-day intervals, up to 6 mg to 10 mg daily in three divided doses at mealtime.

Drug-induced extrapyramidal disturbances

Adults: (initially) 1 mg (taken orally), followed by, if needed, after several hours, up to 15 mg daily; usual dose range is 5 mg to 15 mg daily.

SIDE EFFECTS

Common: Dizziness; nervousness; dry mouth, (mild) nausea; blurred vision; constipation; sensitivity to the sun; painful urination; urinary retention.

Uncommon: Orthostatic hypotension; euphoria; numbness in the hands or feet; sore mouth and tongue; unusual excitement (in high doses).

ADVERSE REACTIONS

Confusion; eye pain; skin rash.

DRUG INTERACTION

With amantadine, increases anticholinergic reactions.

OVERDOSAGE

If any of the following symptoms develops, notify your physician immediately: Hallucinations; mood changes; seizures; (severe) drowsiness; rapid heartbeat; flushing of the skin.

Comments: ARTANE is one of the drugs given to patients who are experiencing severe extrapyramidal symptoms (such as muscle rigidity, tremors, and uncoordinated movements) as a result of another psychiatric drug.

Avoid alcohol while taking this drug; it could increase sedation. Do not take this drug with meals; it might cause nausea or stomach upset. Be careful if driving a car or operating any machinery that requires alertness and good coordination, as the drug is sedating. Sugarless gum or ice chips may relieve the symptom of dry mouth.

Any urinary retention, especially in older men, should be reported to a doctor. If you are over the age of forty, your eyes should be checked periodically for any changes; if you experience any pain in them, notify your doctor.

Pregnancy: Category C (see sidebar on page 69). This means that whatever risk the drug could conceivably pose for the fetus is outweighed by the possible benefits of the drug to the mother. However, you are advised to avoid its use during the first trimester of a pregnancy, whenever possible. (One of its adverse reactions is a false-positive result on a pregnancy test.)

Brand Name
SYMMETREL

Generic Name
amantadine (a-MAN-
ta-deen)

HOW THE DRUG WORKS

Prevents the influenza A virus from reaching susceptible cells, but this drug's precise action in the treatment of parkinsonism or extrapyramidal symptoms is unclear.

PURPOSE

Parkinsonism; drug-induced extrapyramidal reactions.

DOSAGE

Treatment of parkinsonism
Adults: (initially) 100 mg (taken orally) daily, followed, if needed, by increases up to 400 mg daily in divided doses.

Drug-induced extrapyramidal disturbances
Adults: (initially) 100 mg (taken orally), followed, if needed, by increases up to 300 mg daily in divided doses.

SIDE EFFECTS

Common: Dizziness; nausea; constipation; insomnia; loss of appetite; difficulty concentrating; irritability.
Uncommon: Blurred vision; dry mouth and nose; headache; skin rash or purplish-red blotchy spots; fatigue; vomiting.

ADVERSE REACTIONS

Confusion; hallucinations; mood changes; difficult urination; fainting. *Rare:* slurred speech; sore throat or fever; rolling of the eyes; weight gain; edema; shortness of breath.

DRUG INTERACTION

None significant.

OVERDOSAGE

If any of the following symptoms develops, notify your physician immediately: Severe confusion; seizures; severe nightmares or insomnia; hypotension; aggressive behavior.

Comments: SYMMETREL is one of the drugs given to patients who are experiencing severe extrapyramidal symptoms (such as muscle rigidity, tremors, and uncoordinated movements) as a result of another psychiatric drug. Any adverse reactions should be reported to your doctor immediately. People over sixty-five may be more susceptible to symptoms such as confusion, orthostatic hypotension (e.g., dizziness when changing position), and difficulties in urination. For these and other reasons, the elderly should not receive more than 100 mg daily and, perhaps, in divided doses as well.

The drug is best absorbed if taken after meals; it should also be taken several hours before bedtime if insomnia becomes a problem.

Pregnancy: Category C (see sidebar on page 69). This means that whatever risk the drug could conceivably pose for the fetus is outweighed by the possible benefits of the drug to the mother. However, you are advised to avoid its use during the first trimester of a pregnancy, whenever possible. (One of its adverse reactions is a false-positive result on a pregnancy test.)

———————

Brand Name	*Generic Name*
COGENTIN	benztropine (BENZ-tro-peen)

HOW THE DRUG WORKS

By blocking the central cholinergic receptors, this drug helps to control the chemical imbalance that causes the symptoms of parkinsonism.

PURPOSE

Parkinsonism; drug-induced extrapyramidal disturbances.

DOSAGE

Drug-induced extrapyramidal disturbances

Adults: (initially) 1 mg to 2 mg (taken orally) daily, in divided doses; after one to two weeks, the drug may be withdrawn temporarily to determine whether it should be continued or discontinued.

SIDE EFFECTS

Common: Dizziness; nervousness; dry mouth; (mild) nausea; blurred vision; constipation; sensitivity to the sun; painful urination; urinary retention.

Uncommon: Orthostatic hypotension; euphoria; numbness in hands or feet; sore mouth and tongue; unusual excitement (in high doses).

ADVERSE REACTIONS

Confusion; eye pain; skin rash.

DRUG INTERACTION

With amantadine, phenothiazines, and tricyclic antidepressants, it increases anticholinergic reactions.

OVERDOSAGE

If any of the following symptoms develops, notify your physician immediately: Hallucinations; mood changes; seizures; (severe) drowsiness; rapid heartbeat; flushing of the skin.

Comments: COGENTIN is one of the drugs given to patients who are experiencing severe extrapyramidal symptoms (such as muscle rigidity, tremors, and uncoordinated movements) as a result of another psychiatric drug.

Avoid alcohol while taking this drug; it could increase sedation. Do not take it with meals; it might cause nausea or stomach upset. Be careful if driving a car or operating any machinery that requires alertness and good coordination, as the drug is sedating. Sugarless gum or ice chips may relieve the symptom of dry mouth.

Intermittent constipation, distention, or abdominal pain should be reported to your doctor. If any urinary retention occurs, especially in older men, it should also be reported to a doctor.

Pregnancy: Category C (see sidebar on page 69). This means that whatever risk the drug could conceivably pose for the fetus is outweighed by the possible benefits of the drug to the mother. However, you are advised to avoid its use during the first trimester of a pregnancy, whenever possible. (One of its adverse reactions is a false-positive result on a pregnancy test.)

PSYCHOSTIMULANTS

Stimulants have always been part of the repertoire of therapeutic drugs. Of the three drugs under discussion here, methylphenidate was introduced in 1956, and the other two drugs were introduced more recently. They stimulate the sympathetic (*alerting*) nervous system whose neurotransmitter is norepinephrine. Additionally fenfluramine acts on the serotonin system.

Historically used as antidepressants and anorexiants, these drugs have been replaced by newer, more specific, benign medications because of their dependent liabilities and side effects. As a group they now play a secondary or ancillary role, augmenting the effects of conventional antidepressants. However, methylphenidate and pemoline still play a role in the treatment of childhood/adolescent behavior problems.

Action of the Drug

These select stimulants vary in their period of effectiveness. CY-
LERT may not show any significant results for three to four weeks.

Potential Risks

Psychostimulants have some risks associated with their use, and
some people are at greater risk than others.

Children These stimulants should not be used in children
under the age of twelve, except under medical supervision.

Women The safety of all these drugs for use during pregnancy has not been established. However, they can be used *if* the
need is clear *and* the potential benefits outweigh the probable risks
to the fetus. Speak to your physician about its use during pregnancy and if you intend to breast-feed.

Tolerance

The drugs may lose their effectiveness within a few weeks. When
that occurs, you should stop using these drugs. Do *not* increase
their dosage.

Withdrawal

Since these drugs have abuse potential, it is recommended that
they be used for short periods (usually not more than three
months). The exception is DEXEDRINE, which should probably be
used for no more than four weeks. If these drugs are abruptly
stopped after long-term use or high-dose therapy, you may experience symptoms such as depression, fatigue, and insomnia. Even if
you taper the use of the drug, you may experience a little irritability, sleeplessness, or nervousness for a few days.

Side Effects

The frequency and severity of side effects depends on factors such
as the strength of the dose, how long someone has taken the drug,
and (of course) the susceptibility of the user. (See "People at
Particular Risk," page 66.)

Physiological Effects of Stimulants
Behavioral Excitement; anxiety; nervousness; tension; aggressiveness; confusion; insomnia.

Blood system Abnormally low blood-sugar levels.

Circulatory system Heart palpitations; rapid pulse; orthostatic hypotension (dizziness when standing or changing position suddenly); irregular heart rhythms; chest pain.

Dermatological Rash; hives; hair loss; flushing; sweating.

Digestive system Nausea; vomiting, constipation; diarrhea; stomach cramps; rectal gas; difficulty swallowing.

Head and eyes Blurred vision; eye irritation.

Nervous system Headaches; weakness.

Urinary and reproductive system Sexual problems; irregular menstrual cycles.

Other Fever; dry mouth; unpleasant taste.

Guidelines for Use

May cause dry mouth and constipation. Parents must also understand that these drugs can be used only under strict pediatric supervision because of their potential adverse effects on the child's developmental symptoms, specifically, weight gain and growth.

PSYCHOSTIMULANTS

Brand Name	Generic Name
DEXEDRINE	dextroamphetamine (dex-tro-am-FET-a-meen)
RITALIN	methylphenidate (meth-ill-FEN-i-date)
CYLERT	pemoline (PEM-o-lin)
PONDIMIN	fenfluramine (fen-FLURE-a-meen)

PSYCHOSTIMULANTS

Brand Name
DEXEDRINE

Generic Name
dextroamphetamine
(dex-tro-am-FET-
a-meen)

HOW THE DRUG WORKS

By liberating the release of the neurotransmitter norepinephrine, this drug causes an increased wakefulness, alertness, and attention span.

PURPOSE

Attention-deficit disorder (characterized by restlessness, distractibility, and impulsive behavior in abnormally hyperactive children); narcolepsy (sudden attacks of daytime sleep); augment treatment of depression.

DOSAGE

Treatment of attention-deficit disorder
Children three to five years: (initially) 2.5 mg daily, followed by weekly increments of 2.5 mg daily until desired results are reached.
Children six to twelve years: (initially) 5 mg once or twice a day, followed by weekly increments of 5 mg daily until desired results are reached.

Treatment of narcolepsy
Adults: 5 mg to 60 mg (taken orally) in divided doses.
Children over twelve years: (initially) 10 mg daily, followed by weekly increments of 10 mg daily until desired results are reached.
Children six to twelve years: (initially) 5 mg once or twice a day, followed by weekly increments of 5 mg daily until desired results are reached.

SIDE EFFECTS

Common: Irritability; nervousness; restlessness; insomnia.
Uncommon: Blurred vision; decreased sexual desire; constipation; diarrhea; dizziness; dry mouth; nausea; stomach cramps; excessive sweating; unexplained weight loss.

ADVERSE REACTIONS

Rapid heartbeat; inhibits growth and weight gain (in children). *Rare:* chest pain; rash; dyskinesia.

DRUG INTERACTION

Phenothiazine, haloperidol, ammonium chloride, and ascorbic acid (large doses of vitamin C) weaken the effectiveness of the drug.

Antacids, sodium bicarbonate, and acetazolamide increase the effectiveness of the drug.

With MAO inhibitors, it may cause a sudden and dangerous rise in blood pressure.

OVERDOSAGE

If any of the following symptoms develops, notify your physician immediately: Restlessness; tremors; rapid breathing; confusion; hallucinations; panic; depression; seizures; coma.

Comments: First introduced in 1944, DEXEDRINE has enjoyed many street names, the most popular being *uppers* and *speed*. A drawback is its high *dependence-liability*. Over time a psychological and physical dependency may develop, especially in people with a history of drug addiction. For this reason, prolonged use is discouraged and, then, only at the lowest dosage. It should not be used (1) to prevent fatigue, (2) as a first-line treatment of obesity, and rarely, if ever, (3) as an appetite depressant.

When prescribed for hyperactive children, the drug should not be scheduled for an indefinite period; furthermore, it should be interrupted periodically to assess the child's condition.

This drug may produce withdrawal symptoms such as excitement, headache, irritability, nausea, puffing of the cheeks, chewing movements, and wormlike movements of the tongue. It should also be discontinued if weight loss is significant. While taking this drug, avoid drinking coffee or tea; the caffeine will increase the effects of the drug. To avoid insomnia, take the drug at least six hours before bedtime. Sugarless gum or ice chips may relieve the symptom of dry mouth.

Pregnancy: Category C (see sidebar on page 69). This means that whatever risk the drug could conceivably pose for the fetus is outweighed by the possible benefits of the drug to the mother. However, you are advised to avoid its use during the first trimester of a pregnancy, whenever possible.

Brand Name	*Generic Name*
RITALIN	methylphenidate (meth-ill-FEN-i-date)

HOW THE DRUG WORKS

By liberating the release of the neurotransmitter norepinephrine, this drug causes an increased wakefulness, alertness, and attention span.

PURPOSE

Attention-deficit disorder (in abnormally hyperactive children); narcolepsy (sudden attacks of daytime sleep); augment the treatment of depression.

DOSAGE

Treatment of attention-deficit disorder
Children six years and older: (initially) 5 mg to 10 mg daily, given before breakfast and lunch, followed by weekly increments of 5 mg to 10 mg as needed, up to 60 mg daily; if there is no improvement after one month, discontinue the drug.

Treatment of narcolepsy
Adults: (initially) 20 mg to 30 mg daily in divided doses, usually thirty to forty-five minutes before meals; the dosage varies with the patients: some patients require 10 mg to 15 mg daily, while others require 40 mg to 60 mg daily.

SIDE EFFECTS

Common: Loss of appetite (especially in children); nervousness; insomnia (especially in children).

Uncommon: Drowsiness; dizziness; nausea; stomach pain (especially in children).

ADVERSE REACTIONS

Rapid heartbeat; chest pain; skin rash; dyskinesia; fever. *Rare:* Blurred vision; seizures; sore throat and fever. *Long-term use:* Mood changes; unusual weight loss.

DRUG INTERACTION

Increases the effects of anticonvulsants, tricyclic antidepressants, and oral anticoagulants.
Decreases the effects of centrally acting hypertensive drugs.

With MAO inhibitors, it may cause a sudden and dangerous rise in blood pressure.

OVERDOSAGE

If any of the following symptoms develops, notify your physician immediately: Agitation; confusion; vomiting; tremors; muscle twitching; convulsions; euphoria; sweating; rapid breathing; hallucinations; seizures.

Comments: The rule or conventional wisdom concerning the medication of hyperactive children is *prudence.* RITALIN should not be prescribed for an indefinite period. It should be periodically interrupted to assess the child's condition and it usually should be discontinued after puberty. For adults and children alike, the drug should be taken before 6 P.M. because it can cause insomnia, particularly in capsule form (RITALIN-SR).

A drawback is its dependency-liability. Over time a psychological and physical dependency may develop, especially in people with a history of drug addiction. For this reason, prolonged use is discouraged and, then, only at the lowest dosage. It should not be used to prevent fatigue.

This drug may produce withdrawal symptoms such as excitement, headache, irritability, nausea, puffing of the cheeks, chewing movements, and wormlike movements of the tongue. While taking this drug, avoid drinking coffee or tea; the caffeine will increase the effects of the drug. Sugarless gum or ice chips may relieve dry mouth.

Pregnancy: Category C (see sidebar on page 69). This means that whatever risk the drug could conceivably pose for the fetus is outweighed by the possible benefits of the drug to the mother. However, you are advised to avoid its use during the first trimester of a pregnancy, whenever possible.

Brand Name	*Generic Name*
CYLERT	pemoline (PEM-o-lin)

HOW THE DRUG WORKS

By liberating the release of the neurotransmitter norepinephrine, this drug causes an increased wakefulness, alertness, and attention span.

PURPOSE

Attention-deficit disorder with hyperactivity in children.

DOSAGE

Treatment of attention-deficit disorder
Children six years and older: (initially) 37.5 mg daily, given in a single morning dose, followed by weekly increments of 18.75 mg daily as needed; do not exceed 112.5 mg daily; usual dosage is 56.25 mg to 75 mg daily.

SIDE EFFECTS

Common: Loss of appetite; unusual weight loss; insomnia.
Uncommon: Drowsiness; dizziness; nausea; stomachache; increased irritability; depression.

ADVERSE REACTIONS

Nervousness; rapid or pounding heartbeat; seizures; hallucinations; diarrhea.

DRUG INTERACTION

Changes the effectiveness of insulin and oral hypoglycemics.

OVERDOSAGE

If any of the following symptoms develops, notify your physician immediately: Agitation; confusion; vomiting; tremors; hallucinations; severe headache; muscle twitching; euphoria; seizures; unusually large pupils.

Comments: The therapeutic effects of CYLERT may not be evident until three or four weeks' use. Most of the side effects that occur during this period are mild. If side effects persist, however, notify your doctor. The medicine should be taken at least six hours before bedtime to avoid sleep interference.

Although it is structurally dissimilar to DEXEDRINE and RITALIN, CYLERT can produce some of the same adverse reactions. It is also more habit-forming than previously thought. Finally, once this drug is discontinued, the child may experience depression or fatigue for a short period of time, depending upon the amount of medicine taken and how long it was used.

Pregnancy: Category B (see sidebar on page 69). This means that the risk to the fetus is relatively low.

Brand Name	*Generic Name*
PONDIMIN	fenfluramine (fen-FLURE-a-meen)

HOW THE DRUG WORKS

By stimulating an area of the brain (hypothalamus), this drug may affect the sympathetic and parasympathetic nervous systems; it also has serotonin-depleting properties.

PURPOSE

Short-term use as part of a weight-reduction program; also used for certain childhood behavioral disorders.

DOSAGE

Treatment of exogenous obesity and to augment antidepressants
Adults: (initially) 20 mg daily in divided doses, given with meals; maximum dosage 40 mg in divided doses.

SIDE EFFECTS

Common: Diarrhea; drowsiness; dry mouth.
Uncommon: Blurred vision; constipation; unsteadiness; difficult urination; difficulty in speech; headache; irritability; nausea; restlessness; stomach cramps or pain; insomnia or nightmares; pounding heartbeat; unusual sweating; fatigue; diminished sexual drive.

ADVERSE REACTIONS

Confusion; depression; chronic sleep loss; irritability; skin rash or hives; fever; psychosis.

DRUG INTERACTION

Increases the effects of alcohol and CNS depressants.
Decreases the effects of centrally acting hypertensive drugs.

With MAO inhibitors, it may cause a sudden and dangerous rise in blood pressure.

OVERDOSAGE

If any of the following symptoms develops, notify your physician immediately: Extreme nervousness; euphoria; changes in perception.

Comments: Since PONDIMIN has an abuse potential, it should be used only for short periods. Since it can also lose its effectiveness in as little as a few weeks, this drug should be discontinued at the first sign of its ineffectiveness; but do *not* increase its dosage. In some instances, it has been used with success for months, but it should *not* be used longer than six months.

If used longer than two weeks, this drug should not be stopped abruptly, as this might cause acute depression. To avoid withdrawal symptoms such as depression, extreme fatigue, and nightmares, gradually reduce the dosage over one week.

While taking this drug, avoid drinking coffee or tea; the caffeine will increase the effects of the drug. Sugarless gum or ice chips may relieve dry mouth.

Pregnancy: Category C (see sidebar on page 69). This means that whatever risk the drug could conceivably pose for the fetus is outweighed by the possible benefits of the drug to the mother. However, you are advised to avoid its use during the first trimester of a pregnancy, whenever possible.

ANTIANXIETY AGENTS

For the many people who suffered from the debilitating effects of stress and anxiety, the introduction of antianxiety drugs in the 1960s was great news. These drugs were the first medications to therapeutically offer patients effective relief from their symptoms. Prior to the appearance of antianxiety drugs, barbiturates were often used for anxiety relief, but they were considered unsatisfactory because they were far too addicting for people to use for any period of time. These newer antianxiety drugs, designed to treat specific problems of mood, were thought to be less dependent-liable (*addictive*).

Unfortunately, these early drugs were also found wanting. They were so sedating that people could not be comfortable while working a normal day, and these drugs were also found to be alarmingly dependent-liable. By the mid-1970s, there was a dramatic overall decrease in the professional use of all antianxiety drugs, generally, because of a somewhat exaggerated fear of their dependency and habituation.

How these drugs work is not fully clear, but it is believed that the benzodiazepine antianxiety drugs effectively diminish anxiety by decreasing the activity of certain parts of the brain, called the limbic system. It is thought that by adjusting the activity of one of the most abundant inhibitory neurotransmitters in the brain, gaba-ergic, anxiety is reduced.

These drugs not only work to diminish anxiety, especially anxiety associated with depression, but they are also used for musculoskeleton spasms due to muscle or joint inflammation or trauma, or for the withdrawal from other drugs, such as alcohol, panic attacks, or in anesthesia to induce anesthesia. One drug is used to manage anxiety, tension, agitation, and irritability in older patients, including the anxiety associated with alcohol withdrawal; a second treats tremor or delirium tremens (DTs); and a third is used for the management of seizures (with other drugs).

Hypothetically, short-acting benzodiazepines can be used for the treatment of short-term insomnia, but generally they should be used only in those instances in which the sleeplessness is anxiety-based.

Though they are highly sedating—they can decrease the level of consciousness, cause drowsiness, and intellectual impairment, and in some instances decrease motor coordination and impair memory or recall—they have a high therapeutic index. This means that the ratio between their value and their liability is such that, if used correctly, they are quite safe and effective.

Course of Treatment

In general, these drugs take effect almost immediately, especially the short-acting medications. Because of their efficacy and relative safety, these drugs can be used in a variety of circumstances involving treatment of anxiety disorders, including the short-term relief of the anxiety symptoms, such as those associated with airline travel. On the other hand, they are inappropriate for ordinary use, and should not be used to treat the tension of everyday life.

Because of their high dependence-liability, these drugs are seldom used long-term. It is only under closely supervised circumstances that any of these medications should be used as a maintenance drug.

Potential Risks

Antianxiety drugs have some risks associated with their use, and some people are at greater risk than others.

Children Children should receive only the smallest doses of benzodiazepines.

Women Studies have shown that these drugs pose a threat to the fetus. Hence, they should be used during pregnancy *only* if clearly needed and if the benefits outweigh the possible risks. Do not breast-feed while taking benzodiazepines, as they appear in breast milk.

Elderly The elderly should receive only the smallest doses of benzodiazepines.

Dependency

Drug dependence comes in two forms. The first is *dose-related:* the more you take of the drug, the greater the risk of dependence. The second is *time-dependent:* the longer the body is exposed to the drug, the greater the risk of dependence.

Withdrawal

Withdrawal symptoms can begin on the first day you stop or not until the tenth day, and they can last from a week to a month. They are more likely to occur if the antianxiety drug is short-acting, used consistently for more than three months in high dosages, and stopped abruptly. Typical withdrawal symptoms are tremulousness, sweating, sensitivity to the sun, difficulty sleeping, and cramps. More serious forms of withdrawal symptoms are seizures or psychosis. Even if you have used the drug for only two months and tapered its use before stopping, you may experience some irritability, sleeplessness, or nervousness for several days.

Side Effects

The frequency and severity of side effects depend on factors such as the strength of the dose, how long someone has taken the drug, and (of course) the susceptibility of the user. (See "People at Particular Risk," page 66.)

Physiological Effects of Antianxiety Drugs

Behavioral Confusion; depression; drowsiness; dizziness; insomnia; crying; restlessness; behavior changes.

Blood system Abnormal blood counts.

Circulatory system Heart palpitations; irregular heartbeat; changes of blood pressure.

Dermatological Rash; hives; hair loss; itching; yellowing of the skin.

Digestive system Stomach upset; nausea; vomiting, constipation; diarrhea; dry mouth; loss of appetite.

Eyes, ears, and nose Sensitivity to light; blurred vision; double vision; decreased hearing; nasal congestion.

Liver Abnormal liver-function tests.

Nervous system Headaches; lethargy; delirium; fever; vivid dreams.

Urinary and reproductive systems Difficult urination; urine retention; changes in sex drive; menstrual problems.

Other Hiccups; sore gums; ankle and facial swelling.

Guidelines for Use

Do not exceed prescribed doses, nor take the drug longer than prescribed. Its dependent-liabilities make it *habit-forming*. These drugs are not to be used with Macrolide Anti-infectives, e.g., erythromycin, troleandomycin (TAO), clarithromycin (BIAXIN), and azithromycin (ZITHROMAX) as they will raise the level of the drug in the blood and increase the likelihood of side effects.

Avoid using antacids; they may impair absorption of these drugs. While taking these drugs, do not drink alcohol or take other medicines (such as antihistamines) that cause drowsiness.

When using these medications, be extremely careful if you are driving a car or using machinery that requires alertness or good coordination.

ANTIANXIETY AGENTS

LONG-ACTING BENZODIAZEPINES

Brand Name	Generic Name
VALIUM	diazepam (dye-AZ-e-pam)
LIBRIUM	chlordiazepoxide (klor-dye-az-e-POX-ide)

PRO DRUGS

Brand Name	Generic Name
TRANXENE	chlorazepate (klor-AZ-e-pate) dipotassium
CENTRAX	prazepam (PRAZ-e-pam)
PAXIPAM	halazepam (hal-AZ-e-pam)

SHORT-ACTING BENZODIAZEPINES

Brand Name	Generic Name
XANAX	alprazolam (al-PRAZ-oh-lam)
ATIVAN, LORAZ, ALZAPEM	lorazepam (lor-AZ-e-pam)
SERAX	oxazepam (ox-AZ-e-pam)

SHORT-ACTING NONSPECIFIC

Brand Name	Generic Name
INDERAL	propranolol (pro-PRAN-oh-lol)
CATAPRES	clonidine (KLOE-ni-deen)
BUSPAR	buspirone (BOOS-peer-rown)

OBSOLETE DRUGS

Brand Name
EQUANIL, MILTOWN,
MEPROSPAN,
NEURAMATE,
SEDABAMATE,
TRANMEP

Generic Name
meprobamate (me-pro-
BA-mate)

LONG-ACTING BENZODIAZEPINES

Brand Name
VALIUM

Generic Name
diazepam (dye-AZ-
e-pam)

HOW THE DRUG WORKS

Depresses the central nervous system (CNS) at certain areas (limbic) of the brain and reduces anxiety by promoting gaba-ergic transmission at the gaba-benzodiazepine complex of the brain.

PURPOSE

Relief of mild to moderate anxiety and nervous tension; relief of skeletal muscle spasm; acute alcohol-withdrawal syndrome.

Treatment of anxiety disorders and short-term anxiety
Adults: 2 mg to 10 mg (taken orally) daily in divided doses; or 15 mg to 30 mg of extended-release capsules once daily.

Treatment of acute alcohol-withdrawal syndrome
Adults: (first twenty-four hours) 10 mg (taken orally) over first twenty-four hours or as tolerated; then 5 mg daily, in divided doses, as needed, over a five- to seven-day period.

Treatment of skeletal muscle spasms
Adults: 2 mg to 10 mg (taken orally) daily, in divided doses, as needed.
Children: Age and weight of child are critical to determine dose.

SIDE EFFECTS

Common: Dizziness; drowsiness; light-headedness; unsteadiness; hangover.

Uncommon: stomachache; constipation; nausea; watery mouth; slurred speech.

ADVERSE REACTIONS

Skin rash and itching; menstrual irregularities; trouble sleeping; labored breathing; unusual tiredness or weakness; confusion; jaundice.

DRUG INTERACTION

Increases the effects of drugs such as alcohol and other CNS depressants; narcotic analgesics; sedative-hypnotics.

With cimetidine, it increases or prolongs the sedation of this drug.

With fluvoxamine (LUVOX), may cause a marked elevation of VALIUM blood levels.

OVERDOSAGE

If any of the following symptoms develops, notify your physician immediately: Excessive sleepiness; confusion; poor coordination; dizziness; coma.

Comments: Developed in 1963 (one of the oldest of the antianxiety drugs), VALIUM breaks down or metabolizes into two drugs which themselves are active. Hence, this drug has a tendency to accumulate and remain in the body for a long time. Because this buildup can lead to rapid dependence, it is not recommended that the drug be used for more than four months, except under exceptional circumstances. It also can cause short-term functional impairment, especially in the elderly, whose metabolism may be slowed by age.

As with all benzodiazepines, withdrawal symptoms may occur after as little as four to six weeks' use. Because of its long action, any signs of dependence and withdrawal—especially if the drug is stopped abruptly—are often delayed. For example, signs of withdrawal may not occur until five to twelve days after discontinuing the drug and, then, they may last for days or weeks. Withdrawal symptoms include anxiety, irritability, insomnia, psychotic behavior, hallucinations, and severe muscle cramps.

Withdrawal from this long-acting drug is done by tapering, using a short-acting member of the same benzodiazepine family, such as XANAX, or using a nonspecific antiseizure medication, such as TEGRETOL. Any discontinuation of the drug should also be supervised by a doctor.

Like other members of this drug family, VALIUM can cause paradoxical excitement, agitation, and violent behavior. In other words, it may *produce* the type of reaction that the drug was designed to *diminish* or *prevent.* If VALIUM is used in place of an addictive use of alcohol, it can become highly habit-forming.

Pregnancy: Category D (see sidebar on page 69). This means that studies in pregnant women have shown a significant risk to the fetus. Therefore, the drug should be used only if needed in a serious disease and when other, safer drugs have proven to be ineffective or cannot be used.

Brand Name	*Generic Name*
LIBRIUM (capsules)	chlordiazepoxide (klor-dye-az-e-POX-ide)

HOW THE DRUG WORKS

Depresses the CNS at certain areas (limbic) of the brain and reduces anxiety by promoting gaba-ergic transmission at the gaba-benzodiazepine complex of the brain.

PURPOSE

Relief of mild to moderate anxiety disorder and anxiety symptoms; preoperative apprehension and anxiety; withdrawal symptoms of acute alcoholism.

DOSAGE

Treatment of anxiety disorders and anxiety symptoms

Adults: (mild to moderate) 5 mg to 10 mg (taken orally) daily in divided doses; (severe) 20 mg to 25 mg daily in divided doses.

Children over six years: 5 mg daily in divided doses, up to 10 mg, if needed.

Treatment of acute alcohol-withdrawal syndrome

Adults: 50 mg to 100 mg (taken orally) daily in divided doses, up to 300 mg; once agitation is controlled, reduce by tapering to zero level.

SIDE EFFECTS

Common: Dizziness; drowsiness; light-headedness; unsteadiness; hangover.

Uncommon: stomachache; constipation; nausea; watery mouth; slurred speech.

ADVERSE REACTIONS

Skin rash and itching; menstrual irregularities; trouble sleeping; swelling of the legs or feet; labored breathing; unusual tiredness or weakness; confusion; jaundice.

DRUG INTERACTION

Increases the effects of drugs such as alcohol and other CNS depressants; narcotic analgesics; sedative-hypnotics.

With cimetidine, it increases or prolongs the sedation of this drug.

OVERDOSAGE

If any of the following symptoms develops, notify your physician immediately: Excessive sleepiness; confusion; poor coordination; excitation; dizziness; coma.

Comments: Introduced in 1960, LIBRIUM became the first of the class of benzodiazepines. Besides treating symptoms of anxiety, this drug is also used in combination with antidepressants (such as LIMBITROL) in patients with anxious depression. Since metabolism diminishes with age, the drug will be less effectively absorbed in the elderly. Hence, its dosage should be reduced in the elderly so to avoid a toxic buildup. Also, if you have a history of renal (kidney) disease, the dosage should be reduced since the drug may accumulate in the liver.

Like VALIUM, this drug has a tendency to accumulate and remain in the body for a long time. Because this buildup can lead to rapid dependence, it should not be used for more than four months, except under exceptional circumstances. It also can cause short-term functional impairment, especially in the elderly, whose metabolism may be slowed by age.

As with all benzodiazepines, withdrawal symptoms may occur after as little as four to six weeks' use. Because of its long action, any signs of dependence and withdrawal—especially if the drug is stopped abruptly—are often delayed. For example, signs of withdrawal may not occur until five to twelve days after discontinuing the drug and, then, they may last for days or weeks. Withdrawal symptoms include anxiety, irritability, insomnia, psychotic behavior, hallucinations, and severe muscle cramps.

Withdrawal from this long-acting drug is done by tapering, using a short-acting member of the same benzodiazepine family (such as XANAX) or using a nonspecific antiseizure medication (such as TEGRETOL). Any discontinuation of the drug should also be supervised by a doctor.

Like other members of this drug family, this drug can cause paradoxical excitement, agitation, and violent behavior. In other words, it may produce the type of reactions that the drug was designed to diminish or prevent. It also has a dangerous interaction with alcohol.

Pregnancy: Category D (see sidebar on page 69). This means that studies in pregnant women have shown a significant risk to the fetus. Therefore, the drug should be used only if needed in a serious disease and when other, safer drugs have proven to be ineffective or cannot be used.

PRO DRUGS

Pro drugs are drugs with no pharmaceutical action, but in the process of their metabolism in the body, they break down into active ingredients that are therapeutic. Thus, they are called Pro drugs since the Latin and Greek prefix *pro* means to come before, and, in a sense, these drugs come before the metabolite that is the active agent.

These drugs are composed of the primary metabolites or breakdown products of VALIUM. By going directly to the metabolite, it was thought that these drugs would act faster over a shorter period of time and be less dependent. (The theory is that if we skip the process of the drug metabolism or breakdown and go directly to the therapeutic by-products, the drug might work more quickly and with fewer side effects.) What we learned, however, is that the onset and length of action of these *pro* drugs are pretty much the same as for the primary or parent drugs.

Brand Name	*Generic Name*
TRANXENE	chlorazepate (klor-AZ-e-pate) dipotassium

HOW THE DRUG WORKS

Depresses the central nervous system (CNS) at certain areas (limbic) of the brain and reduces anxiety by promoting gaba-ergic transmission at the gaba-benzodiazepine complex of the brain.

PURPOSE

Relief of anxiety disorder and short-term relief of anxiety symptoms; withdrawal symptoms of acute alcoholism; management of seizures (with other drugs).

Treatment of anxiety disorders and anxiety symptoms

Adults: (initially) 15 mg (taken orally) daily in divided doses; followed by 15 mg to 60 mg in a single daily dose at bedtime or in divided doses.

Treatment of acute alcohol-withdrawal syndrome

Adults: (first day) 30 mg (taken orally) followed by 30 mg to 60 mg in divided doses; (second day) 45 mg to 90 mg in divided doses; (third day) 22.5 mg to 45 mg in divided doses; (fourth day) 15 mg to

30 mg in divided doses; gradually reduce doses to 7.5 mg to 15 mg and discontinue as soon as condition stabilizes.

SIDE EFFECTS

Common: Drowsiness; dizziness; light-headedness; unsteadiness; hangover.

Uncommon: Stomachache; constipation; nausea; watery mouth; slurred speech.

ADVERSE REACTIONS

Skin rash and itching; menstrual irregularities; trouble sleeping; blurred vision; swelling of the legs or feet; nervousness and irritability; confusion.

DRUG INTERACTION

Increases the effects of drugs such as alcohol and other CNS depressants; narcotic analgesics; sedative-hypnotics.

With cimetidine, it increases or prolongs the sedation of this drug.

OVERDOSAGE

If any of the following symptoms develops, notify your physician immediately: Excessive sleepiness; confusion; diminished reflexes; excitation; dizziness; coma.

Comments: Since TRANXENE has a prolonged action, particularly in elderly males, its initial treatment for men over the age of sixty calls for only 7.5 mg to 15 mg daily; increases are made gradually, as needed. If you are significantly overweight, your doctor may increase your dosage, and if you have a history of renal (kidney) disease, your dosage may be reduced.

Because it can lead to rapid dependence, it is not recommended that the drug be used for more than four months, except under exceptional circumstances. As with all benzodiazepines, withdrawal symptoms may occur after as little as four to six weeks' use. Signs of withdrawal may not occur until five to twelve days after one abruptly stops, and then symptoms may last for days or weeks. Any discontinuation of the drug should be supervised, and gradually tapered. Withdrawal symptoms include anxiety, irritability, insomnia, psychotic behavior, hallucinations, and severe muscle cramps.

Like other members of this drug family, it can cause paradoxical excitement, agitation, and violent behavior—the very reactions that the drug was designed to diminish or prevent. It also has a dangerous interaction with alcohol.

Pregnancy: Category C (see sidebar on page 69). This means that whatever risk the drug could conceivably pose for the fetus is outweighed by the possible benefits of the drug to the mother. However, you are advised to avoid its use during the first trimester of a pregnancy, whenever possible.

Brand Name	*Generic Name*
CENTRAX	prazepam (PRAZ-e-pam)

HOW THE DRUG WORKS

Depresses the central nervous system (CNS) at certain areas (limbic) of the brain and reduces anxiety by promoting gaba-ergic transmission at the gaba-benzodiazepine complex of the brain.

PURPOSE

Relief of anxiety disorder and short-term relief of anxiety symptoms.

DOSAGE

Treatment of anxiety disorders and anxiety symptoms
Adults: (initially) 30 mg (taken orally) daily in divided doses; followed up 20 mg to 60 mg daily in divided doses as needed. It can also be given as a single 20-mg dose at bedtime, and can be changed, several days later if needed, to the 20-mg to 40-mg range.

SIDE EFFECTS

Common: Fatigue; dizziness; drowsiness; fainting feeling; poor coordination; hangover.
Uncommon: Stomachache; constipation; dry mouth; nausea.

ADVERSE REACTIONS

Skin rash and itching; menstrual irregularities; trouble sleeping; blurred vision; swelling of the legs or feet; nervousness and irritability; confusion.

DRUG INTERACTION

Increases the effects of drugs such as alcohol and other CNS depressants; narcotic analgesics; sedative-hypnotics.

With cimetidine, it increases or prolongs the sedation of this drug.

OVERDOSAGE

If any of the following symptoms develops, notify your physician immediately: Nausea; vomiting; dizziness; abnormal contraction of the pupils.

Comments: Since CENTRAX has a long half-life with a prolonged action in the elderly, its initial treatment for men over the age of sixty calls for only 10 mg to 15 mg daily in several doses. If you are significantly overweight, your doctor may increase your dosage, but if you have a history of renal (kidney) disease, your dosage may be reduced.

Because it can lead to rapid dependence, it is not recommended that the drug be used for more than four months, except under exceptional circumstances. As with all benzodiazepines, withdrawal symptoms may occur after as little as four to six weeks' use. Signs of withdrawal may not occur until five to twelve days after one abruptly stops and, then, may last for days or weeks. Any discontinuation of the drug should be supervised, and only gradually tapered. Withdrawal symptoms include anxiety, irritability, insomnia, psychotic behavior, hallucinations, and severe muscle cramps. It also has a dangerous interaction with alcohol.

Pregnancy: Category C (see sidebar on page 69). This means that whatever risk the drug could conceivably pose for the fetus is outweighed by the possible benefits of the drug to the mother. However,

you are advised to avoid its use during the first trimester of a pregnancy, whenever possible. _____

Brand Name	*Generic Name*
PAXIPAM	halazepam (hal-AZ-e-pam)

HOW THE DRUG WORKS

Depresses the central nervous system (CNS) at certain areas (limbic) of the brain and reduces anxiety by promoting gaba-ergic transmission at the gaba-benzodiazepine complex of the brain.

PURPOSE

Relief of anxiety disorder and short-term relief of anxiety symptoms.

DOSAGE

Treatment of anxiety disorders and anxiety symptoms
   Adults: (usually) 20 mg to 40 mg (taken orally) daily in divided doses, depending upon the patient's response and severity of the symptoms; optimal range is 80 mg to 160 mg daily.

SIDE EFFECTS

   Common: Dizziness; drowsiness; fainting feeling; poor coordination; hangover.
   Uncommon: Stomachache; constipation; dry mouth; nausea.

ADVERSE REACTIONS

Skin rash and itching; menstrual irregularities; trouble sleeping; blurred vision; swelling of the legs or feet; nervousness and irritability; confusion.

DRUG INTERACTION

Increases the effects of drugs such as alcohol and other CNS depressants; narcotic analgesics; sedative-hypnotics.

With cimetidine, it increases or prolongs the sedation of this drug.

OVERDOSAGE

If any of the following symptoms develops, notify your physician immediately: Nausea; vomiting; dizziness; shakiness; shortness of breath.

Comments: Since PAXIPAM has a long half-life, its initial dosage in the elderly or a debilitated patient should be limited to 20 mg once a day. If you are significantly overweight, your doctor may increase your dosage, but if you have a history of renal (kidney) disease, your dosage may be reduced.

Because it can lead to rapid dependence, it is not recommended that the drug be used for more than four months, except under exceptional circumstances. As with all benzodiazepines, withdrawal symptoms may occur after as little as four to six weeks' use. Signs of withdrawal may not occur until five to twelve days after one abruptly stops and, then, may last for days or weeks. Any discontinuation of the drug should be supervised, and only gradually tapered. Withdrawal symptoms include anxiety, irritability, insomnia, psychotic behavior, hallucinations, and severe muscle cramps. It also has a dangerous interaction with alcohol.

Pregnancy: Category D (see sidebar on page 69). This means that studies in pregnant women have shown a significant risk to the fetus. Therefore, the drug should be used only if needed in a serious disease and when other, safer drugs have proven to be ineffective or cannot be used.

SHORT-ACTING BENZODIAZEPINES

This new type of benzodiazepine is short-acting; that is, these drugs act quickly and leave the body relatively quickly. Consequently, they are safer for those people with liver disease and the elderly since they will not become so drowsy during the day. It was thought, initially, that because of their rapid action and departure from the body, these drugs would have a low dependence profile. Unfortunately, that turns out not to be true. On the contrary, these drugs have proven to have a higher dependence-liability than the longer-acting benzodiazepines.

Brand Name	*Generic Name*
XANAX	alprazolam (al-PRAZ-oh-lam)

HOW THE DRUG WORKS

Depresses the central nervous system (CNS) at certain areas (limbic) of the brain and reduces anxiety by promoting gaba-ergic transmission at the gaba-benzodiazepine complex of the brain.

PURPOSE

Relief of anxiety disorder and short-term relief of anxiety symptoms; may be effective in the treatment of panic disorders.

DOSAGE

Treatment of anxiety disorders and anxiety symptoms
Adults: (usually) 0.25 mg to 0.50 mg (taken orally) daily in divided doses, followed by up to 4 mg daily in divided doses, if needed.

SIDE EFFECTS

Common: Dizziness; drowsiness; fainting feeling; poor coordination; hangover.
Uncommon: Stomachache; constipation; dry mouth; nausea.

ADVERSE REACTIONS

Skin rash and itching; weight gain and weight loss; blurred vision; rigidity; akathisia; insomnia; confusion; anterograde amnesia.

DRUG INTERACTION

Increases the effects of drugs such as alcohol and other CNS depressants; narcotic analgesics; sedative-hypnotics.

Increases the effects of tricyclic antidepressants (imipramine and desipramine).

With cimetidine, it increases or prolongs the sedation of this drug.

With nonsedating antihistamines (e.g., SELDANE and HISMANAL), will cause elevation of drug blood levels.

OVERDOSAGE

If any of the following symptoms develops, notify your physician immediately: Nausea; vomiting; dizziness; shakiness; diminished reflexes; coma.

Comments: XANAX is one of the more commonly used short-acting antianxiety drugs because—since it enters and leaves the body so rapidly—it has a low incidence of prolonged drowsiness (*somnolence*). It also has specific antidepressive and antipanic qualities; this makes it effective with other antidepressants and antipsychotic medications. It should be said that, although this drug has been used effectively to treat anxiety associated with depression, it should *not* be used to treat the anxiety and stress of everyday life.

This drug may produce paradoxical symptoms of mania, excitement, and hostility—symptoms that the drug was designed to diminish or prevent. It also has a dangerous interaction with alcohol. This drug may also cause anterograde memory defects—forgetting events that occur only a few hours after taking the medication.

Stopping the drug abruptly or a sharp reduction in its dosage can lead to withdrawal reactions of anxiety, irritability, and insomnia. Even at low doses, this high-potency drug is extremely seductive (it is so effective that it is hard to give up), often making withdrawal problematic. For these reasons, it should not be used for periods exceeding four months. During the withdrawal period, a doctor may replace this drug with a longer-acting benzodiazepine, such as KLONOPIN.

Pregnancy: Category D (see sidebar on page 69). This means that studies in pregnant women have shown a significant risk to the fetus. Therefore, the drug should be used only if needed in a serious disease and when other, safer drugs have proven to be ineffective or cannot be used.

———————

Brand Name	*Generic Name*
ATIVAN, LORAZ, ALZAPEM	lorazepam (lor-AZ-e-pam)

HOW THE DRUG WORKS

Depresses the central nervous system (CNS) at certain areas (limbic) of the brain and reduces anxiety by promoting gaba-ergic transmission at the gaba-benzodiazepine complex of the brain.

PURPOSE

Relief of anxiety disorder and short-term relief of anxiety symptoms or anxiety symptoms mixed with depressive symptoms.

DOSAGE

Treatment of anxiety disorders and anxiety symptoms
Adults: (usually) 2 mg to 3 mg (taken orally) daily in divided doses, followed by 1 mg to 10 mg, as needed, in divided doses (with the largest before bedtime); usual maintenance dosage is 2 mg to 6 mg daily, in divided doses.

SIDE EFFECTS

Common: Drowsiness; dizziness; fainting feeling; unsteadiness; hangover.
Uncommon: Depression; headache; dry mouth; stomach upset.

ADVERSE REACTIONS

Transient amnesia or memory loss; nausea; visual disturbances.

DRUG INTERACTION

Increases the effects of drugs such as alcohol and other CNS depressants; narcotic analgesics; sedative-hypnotics.

OVERDOSAGE

If any of the following symptoms develops, notify your physician immediately: Excessive sleepiness; confusion; coma.

Comments: Like the other short-acting benzodiazepines, ATIVAN enters and leaves the body rapidly. It generally produces the fewest cumulative effects of all the benzodiazepines and is safe and effective with the elderly. It can be injected intramuscularly for rapid effective relief of anxiety (especially in psychotic patients), in conjunction with HALDOL. ATIVAN also has specific antidepressive and antipanic effects, and it is used with other antidepressants and antipsychotic medications. Although ATIVAN has been used effectively to treat anxiety associated with depression, it should not be used to treat the anxiety or tension of everyday life.

Because of its tendency to develop tolerance and dependence, this drug should not be used for periods exceeding four months. Moreover, stopping the drug abruptly or reducing its dosage sharply can lead to withdrawal reactions of anxiety, irritability, and insomnia. When the drug is to be discontinued, its use should be slowly tapered.

Pregnancy: Category D (see sidebar on page 69). This means that studies in pregnant women have shown a significant risk to the fetus. Therefore, the drug should be used only if needed in a serious disease and when other, safer drugs have proven to be ineffective or cannot be used.

Brand Name
SERAX

Generic Name
oxazepam (ox-AZ-e-pam)

HOW THE DRUG WORKS

Depresses the central nervous system (CNS) at certain areas (limbic) of the brain and reduces anxiety by promoting gaba-ergic transmission at the gaba-benzodiazepine complex of the brain.

PURPOSE

Relief of anxiety disorders and short-term relief of anxiety symptoms; withdrawal symptoms of acute alcoholism.

DOSAGE

Treatment of anxiety disorders and anxiety symptoms
    Adults: (mild to moderate symptoms) 10 mg to 15 mg (taken orally) daily, single dose at bedtime, or in divided doses; (severe symptoms) 15 mg to 30 mg daily.

Treatment of alcohol-withdrawal syndrome
    Adults: 15 mg to 30 mg (taken orally) daily in divided doses.

SIDE EFFECTS

    Common: Dizziness; drowsiness; light-headedness; unsteadiness; hangovers.
    Uncommon: Stomachache; constipation; nausea; slurred speech; dry mouth.

ADVERSE REACTIONS

Skin rash and itching; paradoxical excitement; headaches; transient amnesia or memory loss; edema. *Rare:* jaundice.

DRUG INTERACTION

Increases the effects of drugs such as alcohol and other CNS depressants; narcotic analgesics; sedative-hypnotics.

OVERDOSAGE

    If any of the following symptoms develops, notify your physician immediately: Excessive sleepiness; confusion; poor coordination; excitation; dizziness; coma.

Comments: SERAX has a short to mediate half-life; it remains in the body about twelve hours. As a result, this drug has fewer accumulative effects than most other benzodiazepines, including dependency and withdrawal symptoms.

Lower doses are prescribed in those instances of mild to moderate anxiety associated with a major illness. Stronger doses are prescribed for symptoms of severe anxiety or anxiety mixed with depression.

Pregnancy: Category C (see sidebar on page 69). This means that whatever risk the drug could conceivably pose for the fetus is outweighed by the possible benefits of the drug to the mother. However, you are advised to avoid its use during the first trimester of a pregnancy, whenever possible.

SHORT-ACTING NONSPECIFIC

Brand Name	*Generic Name*
INDERAL	propranolol (pro-PRAN-oh-lol)

HOW THE DRUG WORKS

By blocking certain actions of the sympathetic nervous system, this drug lowers oxygen demands of the heart muscle (reducing the occurrence of angina), lowers blood pressure, restricts the renin secretion by the kidneys (lowering blood pressure), and prevents vasodilation of the cerebral arteries (reducing the likelihood of migraine headaches); it also eliminates or diminishes the norepinephrine-caused peripheral symptoms of anxiety.

PURPOSE

Prevention of hypertension (lowers blood pressure); angina pectoris; severe migraine or vascular headaches.

DOSAGE

Treatment of severe migraine headaches

Adults: (usually) 80 mg (taken orally) daily in divided doses, followed by gradual increments of three to seven days up to 240 mg;

usual dosage is 160 mg to 240 mg daily; if symptoms persist after 240 mg for four to six weeks, the drug should be discontinued.

Treatment of short-term (situational) anxiety
  Adults: (usually not a first-line choice) 20 mg in a single dose.

SIDE EFFECTS

Common: Drowsiness; dizziness; fainting feeling; unsteadiness; hangover.
  Uncommon: Depression; headache; dry mouth; stomach upset.

ADVERSE REACTIONS

Transient amnesia or memory loss; nausea; visual disturbances.

DRUG INTERACTION

Increases the effects of drugs such as alcohol and other CNS depressants; narcotic analgesics; sedative-hypnotics.

OVERDOSAGE

  If any of the following symptoms develops, notify your physician immediately: Excessive sleepiness; confusion; coma.

  Comments: INDERAL reduces or eliminates anxiety symptoms such as heart palpitations, sweating, and diarrhea. Because of its fast-acting effects and low dependency, this drug is commonly used for performance anxiety. Other people have found it effective for intense anxiety, such as those moments before boarding an airplane. (Other beta-blockers that are occasionally used for situational anxiety but are not as effective since they are not as fast-acting are TENORMIN, CORGARD, and VISKIN.) However, this drug must be monitored carefully, and it should not be used by people who suffer from asthma or congestive heart failure.

  Pregnancy: Category C (see sidebar on page 69). This means that whatever risk the drug could conceivably pose for the fetus is outweighed by the possible benefits of the drug to the mother. However,

you are advised to avoid its use during the first trimester of a pregnancy, whenever possible.

Brand Name CATAPRES	*Generic Name* clonidine (KLOE-ni-deen)

HOW THE DRUG WORKS

By down-regulating the activity of the central norepinephrine centers, this drug reduces the ability of the sympathetic nervous system to constrict the blood vessels; this results in more relaxed blood vessel walls and lower blood pressure. It also suppresses the peripheral sympathetic effects (such as palpitations) that are characteristic of anxiety.

PURPOSE

Prevention of hypertension (lowers blood pressure); alcohol withdrawal; short-term anxiety.

DOSAGE

Treatment of alcohol and opiate withdrawal
   Adults: (depending upon the severity of the symptoms) 0.1 mg to 2 mg (taken orally) daily.

Treatment of short-term anxiety
   Adults: (used as a single dose in situational anxiety, but its primary use is as an adjunctive medication, sometimes with a major tranquilizer): 0.1 mg to 2 mg (depending upon the severity of the symptoms).

SIDE EFFECTS

Common: Dry mouth; drowsiness; dizziness.
Uncommon: Constipation; insomnia; dry, itching, or burning eyes; vivid dreams; loss of appetite; decreased sexual activity.

ADVERSE REACTIONS

Depression; skin rash and itching; weight gain; hepatitis; urinary retention; congestive heart failure.

DRUG INTERACTION

Increases the effects of drugs such as alcohol and other CNS depressants; narcotic analgesics; sedative-hypnotics.

With propranolol and other beta-blockers, there is a paradoxical rise in blood pressure.

Tricyclic antidepressants and MAO inhibitors may reduce the effectiveness of this drug.

OVERDOSAGE

If any of the following symptoms develops, notify your physician immediately: Profound hypotension; weakness; excessive sleepiness; diminished reflexes; vomiting.

Comments: A powerful antihypertensive designed to reduce high blood pressure, CATAPRES is also an effective antianxiety agent. With prolonged use, however, it may cause lethargy and depression and lose its effectiveness. If discontinued abruptly after prolonged use, this drug can cause withdrawal symptoms such as anxiety, chest pains, insomnia, restlessness, and excessive sweating. If these symptoms occur, see your doctor.

The side effect of dry mouth can be made less troubling with sugarless gum or ice chips.

Elderly patients should be aware that they may continue to feel dizzy when they change positions. They should avoid alcohol while taking this drug.

Pregnancy: Category C (see sidebar on page 69). This means that whatever risk the drug could conceivably pose for the fetus is outweighed by the possible benefits of the drug to the mother. However, you are advised to avoid its use during the first trimester of a pregnancy, whenever possible.

Brand Name	*Generic Name*
BUSPAR	buspirone (BOOS-peer-rown)

HOW THE DRUG WORKS

By interacting with the dopamine, norepinephrine, and serotonin neurotransmitters, this drug relieves anxiety.

PURPOSE

Anxiety disorders and relief of short-term anxiety.

DOSAGE

Treatment of anxiety disorders and short-term anxiety
Adults: (initially) 5 mg (taken orally) daily in divided doses, followed by increases of 5 mg daily every two to three days as needed, up to 60 mg daily; usual dosage is 20 mg to 30 mg given in divided doses.

SIDE EFFECTS

Common: Drowsiness; dizziness; nervousness; nausea; headache; dry mouth; insomnia.

Uncommon: Fatigue; weakness; sweating; light-headedness; confusion; depression.

ADVERSE REACTIONS

Depression; skin rash and itching; weight gain and weight loss; fever; hepatitis; urinary retention; menstrual irregularities; shortness of breath; delayed ejaculation.

DRUG INTERACTION

Increases the effects of drugs such as alcohol and other CNS depressants; narcotic analgesics; sedative-hypnotics.

With MAO inhibitors, this drug may elevate blood pressure.

OVERDOSAGE

If any of the following symptoms develops, notify your physician immediately: Nausea; vomiting; dizziness; drowsiness; stomach upset.

Comments: BUSPAR, the newest of these anxiolytics, is a non-benzodiazepine that relieves anxiety without the side effects common to the benzodiazepines. When BUSPAR has been used in conjunction with PROZAC, it has made the drug less jarring, that is, reduced the likelihood of producing any nervousness with PROZAC. It is only speculated, but BUSPAR may also relieve the sexual side effects caused by SSRI medications, such as PROZAC. Because it is nonsedating, this drug does not interfere with motor coordination or complex tasks. It does not produce tolerance or dependency. On the other hand, people who have previously been treated with benzodiazepines miss the calming, sedating side effect of these drugs. Hence, this drug may appear to be less effective to some people.

Another difference is that this drug may require at least a week of various dosage changes and a great deal of patience between the doctor and the patient in order to find the right dose. Signs of improvement are usually apparent within ten days, but optimal results will take about three to four weeks. It is best to take this drug with food to avoid any stomach upset.

Pregnancy: Category B (see sidebar on page 69). This means that the risk to the fetus is relatively low.

OBSOLETE DRUGS

Brand Name	Generic Name
EQUANIL, MILTOWN, MEPROSPAN, NEURAMATE, SEDABAMATE, TRANMEP	meprobamate (me-pro-BA-mate)

HOW THE DRUG WORKS

By depressing the central nervous system (CNS) at certain areas (limbic) of the brain, this drug reduces anxiety.

PURPOSE

Relief of anxiety disorders and short-term anxiety and nervous tension.

DOSAGE

Treatment of anxiety disorders and short-term anxiety
Adults: 1,200 mg to 1,600 mg (taken orally) daily in divided doses, or up to 2,400 mg daily if needed.
Children six to twelve years: 100 mg to 200 mg daily in divided doses. (Not recommended for children under six years.)

SIDE EFFECTS

Common: Drowsiness; dizziness; light-headedness; unsteadiness.
Uncommon: Stomachache; diarrhea; nausea; slurred speech; upset stomach.

ADVERSE REACTIONS

Skin rash and itching; rapid heartbeat; heart palpitations; unusual bleeding or bruising; chills; hives.

DRUG INTERACTION

Increases the effects of drugs such as alcohol and other CNS depressants; narcotic analgesics; sedative-hypnotics.

OVERDOSAGE

If any of the following symptoms develops, notify your physician immediately: Severe confusion; shortness of breath; staggering; unusually slow heartbeat; severe weakness.

Comments: Introduced in 1955 as an effective muscle relaxant, meprobamate became the first commonly or popularly used tranquilizer. However, this drug was found to be dependent-forming and, if stopped abruptly, withdrawal symptoms would occur. Also, its sedating effects would cause confusion, disorientation, and dizziness, especially in the elderly. For these reasons, this drug is seldom used nowadays.
Withdrawal from this drug should be accomplished gradually, probably over a period of two weeks. The precise length of time needed to withdraw from this drug depends upon the dosage you were taking daily. If the withdrawal is too abrupt, symptoms may

range from confusion, hallucinations, nightmares, and insomnia to seizures.

While taking the drug, be very careful about driving a car or operating machinery that requires alertness and coordination. Avoid alcohol. Take this drug with food to reduce the likelihood of stomach upset.

Pregnancy: Category D (see sidebar on page 69). This means that studies in pregnant women have shown a significant risk to the fetus. Therefore, the drug should be used only if needed in a serious disease and when other, safer drugs have proven to be ineffective or cannot be used.

MOOD STABILIZERS

Lithium, the first of the mood stabilizers (formerly referred to as antimanic or anticonvulsant drugs), was developed and used in a variety of nineteenth-century patent medicines for the treatment of ailments such as arthritis and gout. Its effectiveness in the treatment of manic behavior was discovered only in 1949. An Australian physician named Andrew Cade learned of the therapeutic value of lithium carbonate when he noted its quieting effects on animals. Subsequent experiments demonstrated that the drug calmed patients who were suffering from a variety of psychotic behaviors.

The drug was not immediately accepted in the United States because of its potential toxicity. The drug was prescribed as a salt substitute in the 1950s for people with high blood pressure. Unfortunately, many of these people transferred their craving for salt to this lithium-containing salt substitute and developed lithium poisoning.

By 1970, however, when the drug was approved for use in the United States, its value in safely treating manic behavior was well established. It is now the most commonly used major member of the mood stabilizer (*antimanic*) family of drugs.

Mood-stabilizer drugs are used to treat people who suffer from cyclic mood changes ranging from easy or exaggerated excitement to grandiose and unrealistic views of oneself. These symptoms can also include episodes of depression. The goal of the mood stabilizers is to establish a range of mood and behavior that allows you to function normally.

Course of Treatment
Stages

1. Someone suffering from acute episodes of manic psychosis is first treated with a neuroleptic until the psychosis abates.
2. Then a mood stabilizer is prescribed for a minimum of fourteen days—the latency period for lithium.
3. Once the mood swings have been brought under control, the medication may be continued at the lowest dose during the maintenance period of the drug therapy.

Potential Risks
All mood-stabilizing drugs have some risks associated with their use, and some people are at greater risk than others.

Children   Some of these drugs can be administered to children, but only with reservations. Each drug has different risks for children: KLONOPIN is most sensitive in children, but can be used; the safety of TEGRETOL has not been established for children under six; DEPAKOTE may cause liver problems in children under two; and lithium should not be used in children under twelve. In every instance of drug use, the weight, general health and severity of the child's symptoms are taken into consideration before any of these drugs are prescribed.

Women   Some of these drugs are dangerous to the fetus and should not be used during pregnancy. Other drugs can be used with relative safety, and most mothers receiving mood stabilizers deliver *normal* babies. However, lithium and DEPAKOTE are considered high-risk drugs for pregnant women. (See Pregnancy code for each drug.) If you intend to breast-feed, consult your doctor; these drugs do appear in breast milk.

Elderly   TEGRETOL may be more likely to produce agitation and confusion in the elderly than in younger patients.

Side Effects
The frequency and severity of side effects or adverse reactions depend on factors such as the strength of the dose, how long someone has taken the drug, and the susceptibility of the user. (See "People at Particular Risk," page 66.)

Physiological Effects of Mood Stabilizers
Behavioral   Drowsiness; mood changes; behavioral changes; hallucinations.

Circulatory system   (TEGRETOL) Changes in blood pressure, abnormal heart rhythm; blood clots. (KLONOPIN) Heart palpitations.

Dermatological   Hives; rash; itching; swelling; hair loss. (TEGRETOL) yellowing of the skin or eyes; bruising or bleeding; sensitivity to the sun.

Digestive system   Nausea; vomiting; loss of or increased appetite; constipation; diarrhea.

Head and eyes   Double vision; unusual eye movements; blurred vision; red, itching eyes.

Nervous system   Depression; clumsiness; slurred speech.

Respiratory system   Difficulty swallowing or breathing; (TEGRETOL) pneumonia.

Guidelines for Use
These drugs cause drowsiness, dizziness, and blurred vision. Use caution if you are driving a car or operating machinery that requires alertness or good coordination.

It is best to take these medicines with food—to avoid an upset stomach.

Noncompliant rates run as high as 30 percent to 40 percent in those patients who suffer from both mood and anxiety disorders. Adherence increases among these people, however, when they know more about the illness and the purpose of the drug, have developed various reliable coping mechanisms, and have interpersonal and psychosocial support available.

See your doctor if you experience bleeding or bruising, yellowing of the skin or eyes, dark urine, swelling, fever or chills. Always notify your doctor if the drug causes any side effects that persist for more than a week.

MOOD STABILIZERS

Brand Name	*Generic Name*
LITHIUM CARBONATE	lithium (LITH-e-oom)

LITHIUM SUBSTITUTES

Brand Name	*Generic Name*
TEGRETOL	carbamazepine (kar-ba-MAZ-e-peen)
DEPAKENE	valproic acid (val-PRO-ic acid)
KLONOPIN	clonazepam (clo-NAZ-e-pam)

Brand Name	*Generic Name*
LITHIUM CARBONATE	lithium (LITH-e-oom)

HOW THE DRUG WORKS

By altering the metabolism of norepinephrine and serotonin and, in turn, altering the environment of the cell membrane, this drug stabilizes mood swings.

PURPOSE

Control and prevention of manic episodes of manic-depressive illness; in the treatment of mania along with major tranquilizers (as part of manic-depressive illness); used in cases of depression that do not respond to other medications.

DOSAGE

Prevention or control of mania

Adults: (for long-term control) 900 mg to 1,800 mg daily, in divided doses, depending upon blood level or signs of toxicity. Once stable, the dosage determined can be given as single dose at night.

SIDE EFFECTS

Common: Excessive thirst; increased frequency of urination; slight trembling of the hands.

Uncommon: Skin rash; bloated feeling; slight muscle twitching.

ADVERSE REACTIONS

Feeling faint; irregular pulse; trouble breathing (especially after exercise); rapid heartbeat; fatigue; weight gain. *Rare:* Blue color and pain in the fingers and toes; coldness in the arms and legs; vision problems.

DRUG INTERACTION

With THORAZINE and salts, such as aminophylline, sodium bicarbonate, and sodium chloride (table salt), this drug *decreases* lithium effectiveness by *increasing* its excretion.

With HALDOL or MELLARIL, it causes an encephalopathic syndrome, with tremors and extrapyramidal symptoms.

With NSAID (nonsteroidal anti-inflammatory drugs), will raise the blood level of LITHIUM.

With carbamazepine, probenecid, indomethacin, methyldopa, and piroxicam, it can cause lithium toxicity.

Diuretics increase the reabsorption of lithium; this can increase the risk of toxicity.

OVERDOSAGE

If any of the following symptoms develops, notify your physician immediately: Early signs—Diarrhea; severe drowsiness; abdominal pain; loss of appetite; nausea; trembling; slurred speech. Late signs—Blurred vision; confusion; hypotension; dizziness; seizures; coma.

Comments: If you are on a fasting diet, use diuretics, or suffer from diarrhea, LITHIUM must be used cautiously. The same caution should also be exercised by (1) people who lose a great deal of body salt through excessive vomiting or sweating, or (2) people on sodium-restricted diets or drugs that deplete salt from the body. In all these instances, blood sodium levels fall; this interferes with the excretion of lithium from the body. As a result, concentrations of the drug build up in the body, sometimes to toxic levels. In these situations, your doctor may decrease or curtail your dosage of lithium.

A second caution concerns those women in their first trimester of pregnancy because lithium is associated with a particular form of cardiac abnormality in the fetus. Your doctor may take you off the drug during this period and either replace it with another mood stabilizer or keep you drug-free until your child is born. For these and many other reasons, someone starting a program of lithium use should have an electrocardiogram and thyroid function and kidney function tests prior to using the drug.

If you are taking a diuretic or a nonsteroidal anti-inflammatory drug, your doctor may have to reduce the dosage of LITHIUM in order to maintain proper blood levels in relation to the drug. When taking LITHIUM, a better choice of medications than an NSAID would be ibuprofen (MOTRIN or ADVIL) or naprosyn (ALEVE). LITHIUM use in the elderly may increase their risk of bradycardia, or slow heartbeat.

If excessive thirst continues to be a problem, your doctor may prescribe a diuretic or decrease the amount of the drug. Drinking more water helps. You should drink as much as eight to twelve glasses of water or liquids per day while taking this drug.

Some people fear the drug will adversely affect their kidneys. These apprehensions are highly exaggerated. The incidence of serious or irreversible kidney damage is very small. In all likelihood, your blood levels will be regularly monitored by your doctor to keep them from reaching levels that could harm your kidneys. If your blood levels were to increase periodically and without a change of dose, your doctor would probably reduce your dosage or, eventually, place you on another medication.

Your lithium levels will be monitored once or twice a week for the first three or four weeks, then only once a month for several months. By the sixth month, when the drug should have achieved a steady state in your blood, it will need to be monitored only every one to three months. Most commercial or hospital laboratories do this monitoring on a routine basis.

While taking this drug, a common problem is hand tremor. Your hand may shake periodically, both when it is being used and at rest. These jerky movements may become more vigorous during part of the day and then become relatively mild. It is a nuisance since it makes some daily activities rather difficult, such as drinking from a cup or writing, but no special treatment is usually needed. Again, if it persists, your doctor may treat the side effect with another drug, such as INDERAL.

If you find that the capsule form or carbonate form is irritating to your stomach, your doctor may give you the drug in its liquid form, called LITHIUM CITRATE.

Some doctors have effectively prescribed the drug to treat cluster headaches, premenstrual syndrome (PMS), and eating disorders. It is also asserted that the drug will prevent depression; however, the data are inconclusive.

Pregnancy: Category D (see sidebar on page 69). This means that studies in pregnant women have shown a significant risk to the fetus. Therefore, the drug should be used only if needed in a serious disease and when other, safer drugs have proven to be ineffective or cannot be used.

LITHIUM SUBSTITUTES

For people whose mood swings are not relieved by lithium, or who cannot tolerate its side effects, there are a number of effective substitutes. The first major substitutes are borrowed from the field of neurology: carbamazepine, valproic, and clonazepam. These anticonvulsant medications, normally prescribed in the treatment of seizures, were found to have reliable antimanic or mood-stabilizing effects.

Brand Name	*Generic Name*
TEGRETOL	carbamazepine (kar-ba-MAZ-e-peen)

HOW THE DRUG WORKS

By controlling the activity of the nerve impulses in the brain or CNS, this drug prevents or reduces seizures. (The use of anticonvulsants developed from a theoretical model of manic attacks known as *kindling.* The model argues that the effects of persistent excitability in the limbic system of the brain accumulate until it causes a kind of *affective seizure* known clinically as a manic attack.)

PURPOSE

Maintain mood; prevent or reduce the number of seizures; reduce pain of trigeminal neuralgia; help reduce manic attacks and manic symptoms.

DOSAGE

Prevention or control of seizures

Adults: initially, 200 mg (taken orally) daily in divided doses; (for long-term control) 800 mg to 1,200 mg daily, in divided doses.

Children six to twelve years: initially, 100 mg (taken orally), followed by gradual increases of 100 mg to 1,000 mg daily in divided doses.

Children twelve to seventeen years: initially, 200 mg (taken orally) daily in divided doses, up to 1,000 mg (if needed) in divided doses.

SIDE EFFECTS

Common: Clumsiness, light-headedness; drowsiness; nausea.

Uncommon: Aching muscles; constipation; excessive thirst; increased frequency of urination; slight trembling of the hands.

ADVERSE REACTIONS

Blurred vision; confusion; hostility; seizures; severe nausea. (Less common): Hives; itching; confusion (in the elderly); behavioral changes (in children). *Rare:* Chest pain; slow heartbeat; swelling feet and legs; visual hallucinations; pale stools; sore throat and fever; yellowing of the skin and eyes.

DRUG INTERACTION

Increases the effectiveness of lithium.

Decreases the effectiveness of theophylline, warfarin, phenytoin, doxycycline, haloperidol.

With MAO inhibitors, it produces excitability and seizures.

Phenobarbital and primidone decrease the effectiveness of this drug.

With oral contraceptives, there is breakthrough bleeding.

OVERDOSAGE

If any of the following symptoms develops, notify your physician immediately: Severe dizziness or drowsiness; shallow or slow breathing; seizures; trembling and twitching, convulsions; coma.

Comments: Chemically similar to the antidepressant imipramine, TEGRETOL has been used both with lithium and as an alternative drug for the treatment of manic symptoms associated with episodes of manic-depressive illness. This drug is usually effective within two weeks of taking it. However, a peculiar quality of this drug is that it heightens its own metabolism or breakdown (and that of other drugs, such as oral contraceptives, which makes them less effective). Consequently, every few weeks its dosage has to be raised to maintain effectiveness.

It is not clear what the relationship is between the size of the dose and the likelihood of adverse affects. Generally, the drug is given slowly, with blood levels monitored frequently during the early use of the drug. You must wait fourteen days (or longer) after discontinuing MAO inhibitors before beginning this drug.

A virtue of the drug is that it can be *night-loaded*, that is, all of it can be taken at night. This is especially important for people with severe insomnia. This drug should be taken with milk or at meals to reduce stomach upset, and an increase of daily liquids may minimize the discomfort from constipation.

Pregnancy: Category C (see sidebar on page 69). This means that whatever risk the drug could conceivably pose for the fetus is outweighed by the possible benefits of the drug to the mother. However, you are advised to avoid its use during the first trimester of a pregnancy, whenever possible.

Brand Name	*Generic Name*
DEPAKENE	valproic acid (val-PRO-ic acid)

HOW THE DRUG WORKS

By increasing the levels of a certain neurotransmitter (gamma-aminobutyric or GABA), this drug inhibits the abnormal nerve impulses that produce seizures. (The use of anticonvulsants developed from a theoretical model of manic attacks known as *kindling*. The model argues that the effects of persistent excitability in the limbic system of the brain accumulate until it causes a kind of *affective seizure* known clinically as a manic attack.)

PURPOSE

Stabilizes mood; prevents or reduces the number of simple (petit mal) and complex seizures; reduces the pain of trigeminal neuralgia; helps reduce or prevent manic symptoms.

DOSAGE

Mood stabilizing

Adults: initially, 500 mg (taken orally) daily in divided doses; maximum dosage is based on 20 mg for every kg (2.2 lb) of body weight but not to exceed 2000 mg.

Children six to twelve years: initially, 100 mg (taken orally), followed by gradual increases of 100 mg to 1,000 mg daily in divided doses.

Children twelve to seventeen years: initially, 200 mg (taken orally) daily in divided doses, up to 1,000 mg (if needed) in divided doses.

SIDE EFFECTS

Common: Gastrointestinal distress (indigestion, mild cramps, and diarrhea); increased appetite and weight gain; change in menstrual periods; occasional trembling of the hands and arms.

Uncommon: Constipation; drowsiness; dizziness; depression; irritability.

ADVERSE REACTIONS

Seizures; poor coordination; skin rash; facial swelling; irrational thinking or perceptions; rigid thinking; unusual agitation and excitement; repetitive nonpurposeful movement (e.g., Monty Python's silly walk).

DRUG INTERACTION

Increases the effects of anticoagulants (oral), barbiturates, clonazepam, phenytoin, primidone, and salicylates (e.g., aspirin).

With alcohol or other CNS depressants, it increases its sedating effects.

With CLOZAPINE, will raise level of the drug in the blood.

OVERDOSAGE

If any of the following symptoms develops, notify your physician immediately: Severe drowsiness; unsteadiness; shallow breathing; deep coma.

Comments: A second member of the antiseizure family (sometimes called anticonvulsants), DEPAKENE, also found in a salt form as DEPAKOTE, is used separately and with lithium to treat manic behavior. This drug also helps those individuals who have wide and rapid mood changes from manic to depressive moods or vice versa (so-called *rapid-cycling*).

As in the use of lithium, blood samples and liver tests need to be taken during the first four to six weeks of your use of this drug. Dosages of this drug may be changed because of the results of the blood samples. It is recommended that the drug be used aggressively, that is, it can be prescribed immediately at the dose level assumed to be appropriate for the patient rather than started at a cautiously reduced dose level, because rapid escalation will decrease the agitation and irritability of mania. If the dose level is found to be too high, it can be lowered. Short-term use of DEPAKOTE may be indicated for behavioral control until the cause of the behavior is determined and a more specific treatment is instituted.

Quite the opposite of TEGRETOL, this drug inhibits its own metabolism (and that of other drugs, too). Thus, instead of *increasing* its dosage to maintain effectiveness (as in the case of TEGRETOL), the dosage of DEPAKOTE may be periodically *lowered* to maintain proper blood levels. It is important, therefore, that you do not exceed the recommended dosage or discontinue it abruptly, as this drug may produce adverse reactions.

It is best to take this drug with milk or food to avoid an upset stomach. Do not chew or crush the tablets or capsules, as they may irritate your mouth or throat. If you are taking this drug in its liquid form (tasty red syrup), do not mix it with carbonated beverages; the effervescence may also irritate the mouth and throat. Finally, if you take aspirin on a daily basis, consult with your doctor before starting this drug. Aspirin may increase your bleeding.

Pregnancy: Category D (see sidebar on page 69). This means that studies in pregnant women have shown a significant risk to the fetus. Therefore, the drug should be used only if needed in a serious disease and when other, safer drugs have proven to be ineffective or cannot be used.

———————

Brand Name KLONOPIN	*Generic Name* clonazepam (clo-NAZ- e-pam)

HOW THE DRUG WORKS

By acting on the gaba-benzodiazepine complex of the brain as a neuroinhibitory agent, this drug stabilizes mood.

PURPOSE

Prevents or reduces the number of simple (petit mal) and complex seizures; reduces the pain of trigeminal neuralgia; helps reduce manic symptoms.

DOSAGE

Prevention or control of seizures

Adults: initially, 1.5 mg (taken orally) daily in divided doses, followed by increases of 0.5 mg to 1.0 mg daily every three days until seizures are controlled; maximum dosage is 20 mg daily.

Children up to ten years of age or a weight of at least 30 kilograms/65 pounds: 0.01 mg to 0.03 mg (taken orally) daily, in divided doses, up to 0.05 mg daily; the dosage should be increased by 0.25 mg to 0.5 mg increments every three days, but should not exceed 0.1 mg to 0.2 mg daily.

SIDE EFFECTS

Common: Dizziness; drowsiness; light-headedness; unsteadiness.

Uncommon: Diarrhea; stomachache; constipation; nausea; slurred speech.

ADVERSE REACTIONS

Skin rash or itching; headaches; unusual fatigue or weakness; confusion.

DRUG INTERACTION

Increases the effects of drugs such as alcohol and other CNS depressants and other anticonvulsants.

OVERDOSAGE

If any of the following symptoms develops, notify your physician immediately: Severe drowsiness; confusion; diminished reflexes.

Comments: Its long half-life and rapid onset (*short latency period*) of antimanic activity gives KLONOPIN significant advantages over other mood stabilizers. (It is also an antianxiety drug.) Technically, KLONOPIN is not considered a true mood stabilizer, but it does reduce agitation effectively in people suffering from depression and psychosis. Because of its long half-life, it has been used to withdraw people who are dependent upon the shorter-acting benzodiazepines. However, with extended use, this drug may cause a physical dependence and tolerance of its own, especially in addiction-prone patients. While taking this drug, you will need to have periodic blood samples taken and liver function tests performed.

KLONOPIN should never be discontinued abruptly, or it may precipitate withdrawal symptoms such as hallucinations, trembling, anxiety, vision problems, seizures, nightmares, and other trouble sleeping. Even if you discontinue this drug by tapering its use after a regimen of high doses for an extended period, your body may need an adjustment of two weeks before you are free of all symptoms (for example, hangovers).

It is common to feel drowsy during the day with this drug, so drive a car only with great caution. Avoid alcohol while taking this drug; this could increase sedation.

Pregnancy: Category C (see sidebar on page 69). This means that whatever risk the drug could conceivably pose for the fetus is outweighed by the possible benefits of the drug to the mother. However, you are advised to avoid its use during the first trimester of a pregnancy, whenever possible.

Glossary

Active metabolites: by-products of the drug breaking down in your system. They can be a mixed blessing. Active metabolites are important in medications when a prolonged effect is wanted. For example, because the level of VALIUM in the blood does not fluctuate sharply between doses, it is considered a good maintenance medication.

On the other hand, since active metabolites prolong the drug's stay in the body, repeated doses of a drug increase its effects and the risk of more adverse reactions.

Agranulocytosis: a condition whereby the number of white blood cells (granulocytes) drops to extremely low levels because fewer are produced or more are being destroyed. The symptoms include high fever and ulcers of the mouth, rectum, and vagina. If caused by drug use, the condition is usually reversed within seven to ten days following the discontinuation of the drug.

Agitated depression: depression accompanied by agitation, restlessness, or anxiety (wringing of the hands or moaning). Often it is accompanied by anger and fault-finding, together with feelings of hopelessness.

Amenorrhea: an absence of menstruation caused by pregnancy, active breast-feeding, minor hormonal disturbances, or the possible use of birth-control pills.

Anticholinergic effects: effects that come about as a result of drugs that block the transmission of the neurotransmitter acetylcholine. Common side effects are dry mouth, constipation, and blurred vision. Other less common symptoms are urinary retention, increased or decreased sweating, and increased heart rate.

Arrhythmia: any variation of the normal rhythm of the heartbeat. Most arrhythmias are transitory and harmless, but some are serious and often last a lifetime. This problem can be successfully treated with various cardiac drugs that regulate the heartbeat. Pacemakers can also correct the problem.

    If, however, someone with a history of arrhythmias were to take a drug whose unwanted effects aggravated the problem—these drugs are usually contraindicated, that is, not prescribed to people—this might trigger a heart attack.

Bipolar depression: what we at one time referred to as manic depression. The term describes both poles of mood—depression and mania—and is characterized by the predominant type, such as bipolar manic, bipolar depressive, or bipolar mixed.

Central nervous system (CNS) depression: a condition in which the activity of the nervous system is sufficiently diminished to produce extreme drowsiness, poor muscle coordination, slowed respiration, and possibly coma and death.

Drug interaction: an interaction between two medications given at the same time, altering the effects of one or both drugs, sometimes canceling or magnifying them.

Emergent side effects: side effects that occur after a week or more of drug use, such as fatigue in the patient.

Empirical dose range: the effective dose range arrived at by trial and error, starting with the lowest dose possible.

Endogenous depression: a depression from within or one caused by a biological condition (organic); also referred to as a *major affective disorder*.

Extrapyramidal symptoms (eps): abnormal motor movements that include twitching and involuntary movements of the mouth, hands, and feet; spasms of the neck muscles; severe stiffness of the back muscles; rolling of the eyes; convulsions; and difficulty swallowing. Many of these symptoms resemble those of Parkinson's disease.

(The following is a short glossary of motor movements that fall in the general category of extrapyramidal symptoms.)

Dystonia—a general term for abnormal muscle tone that leads to abnormal positions and distorted twisting of the extremities of the body, including the arms, legs, neck, and head.

Akathisia (acathisia)—a physical restlessness, characterized by an anxious inability to sit still, and often accompanied by a mental restlessness, e.g., *racing thoughts*.

Akinesia—decreased motor movements, including muscle rigidity; slowness of movements; lack of facial expression; drooling; and arresting tremor (which is slow and rhythmic in nature). It can lead to severe overall rigidity: tin-man type.

Dyskinesia—involuntary muscle spasms, especially abnormal movements of the mouth; chewing motions; searching movements of the tongue (often called *catching-flies*); and sucking, licking, and lip-pursing movements. It includes involuntary rhythmic movements of the hands and legs or feet.

Lactorrhea: (*lac* means *milk* in Latin and *rhoia* means *flow* in Greek): the discharge of breast milk between nursings and after weaning the infant. Certain drugs will promote a small inappropriate discharge, but there is no risk to health.

Lowest dosage-range: the smallest dosage (amount of the effective drug) at which the drug will remain effective. The lowest dose is important because side effects are usually dose-related: lower doses yield fewer side effects. A low dose-range is particularly relevant for treating the elderly and the very young.

Major and minor tranquilizers: nontechnical terms by which we can distinguish between the two principal categories of tranquilizers. As would be expected, major tranquilizers are far more powerful than minor tranquilizers. Major tranquilizers are usually used for the treatment of anxiety associated with major disorders, such as psychosis, whereas the less powerful minor tranquilizers are generally used to treat neurotic or characterologic disorders.

Manic-depressive psychosis: noticeable mood swings ranging from normal to elation or depression, or alternating between the two extremes; also referred to as a *bipolar affective disorder*.

Neuroleptic malignant syndrome (NMS): symptoms including muscular rigidity, being dazed and disoriented, sweating profusely, incontinence, high blood pressure, and temperatures as high as 106 degrees Fahrenheit are associated with the use of neuroleptics. Besides discontinuing the medication, treatment usually includes taking (1) plenty of fluids and (2) other drugs that relieve the symptoms. This condition occurs twice as often in males as in females; most patients are over the age of forty. This syndrome seldom occurs outside a hospital.

Nonspecific effects: valued psychiatric or mood-altering effects of drugs that are not *specific* to their original design or intention. Antihistamines, designed to treat histamine responses in people suffering from allergies, are also excellent mild sedatives. INDERAL, an antihypertensive drug devised principally to lower blood pressure, has anxiety-reducing effects.

Obsessive-compulsive disorder: recurrence of images or impulses, or repetitive ritualistic behaviors which someone is compelled to perform. Though recognized as foreign, irrational, and purposeless, any attempt to resist them usually leads to increased anxiety.

Oculogyric crisis: an involuntary rolling or fixation of the eyes upward or an inability to focus; the crisis may last for several minutes or hours.

Orthostatic hypotension: faintness caused by a sudden drop in

blood pressure immediately after standing erect from a lying or
sitting position.

Photosensitivity: easily sunburned.

Priapism: a rare but serious condition whereby blood becomes
trapped in the penis and produces a prolonged erection that is
unrelated to any sexual desire. In addition to blood abnormalities, certain psychiatric drugs can produce this condition.
If you experience priapism, notify your doctor immediately.

Psychotic behavior: behavior—such as profoundly rigid thinking, repetitive nonpurposeful movement, or excitement (unrelated to external stimuli)—associated with a profound disorder
of thinking, mood, and an inability to distinguish what is real
from what is fantasy.

Psychotic depression: severe depression accompanied by fixed
ideas that are inconsistent with reality and often a product of
guilt. Psychotic depression includes symptoms such as fears
that (1) someone has a terrible disease, (2) something is growing inside of them, or (3) their spouse is unfaithful.

Refractory depression: *refractory* means *obstinate* or *stubborn*.
In this case, it characterizes a depression that has resisted ordinary treatment.

Retrograde amnesia: a loss of memory for events and situations
just preceding the time of illness or drug use. In other words,
the drug will cause a memory loss of events both during and
prior to drug use. This phenomenon may strike some people as
alarming, especially the elderly, because they may confuse the
temporary memory loss as evidence of some form of dementia
(e.g., Alzheimer's disease).

Retrograde ejaculation: a process whereby the ejaculate enters
the bladder rather than continuing through the urethra and out
the penis. It is a harmless phenomenon in itself, but it may be an
early sign of sexual dysfunction. It also occurs commonly in
men with diabetes. If it occurs while you are using a psychiatric
drug, and it persists, ask your doctor to change the drug.

Serotonin syndrome: symptoms of confusion, fear, sweating,
clumsiness, erratic eye movement, shivering, and hyperreflexia,

caused by a drug interaction between SSRIs and antidepressants or the addition of a second antidepressant, such as MAO inhibitors, without allowing for a sufficient washout period. Moving from one class of antidepressant to another requires a washout period of five weeks.

Short- and long-acting drugs: *short-acting* drugs act rapidly and leave the body quickly. They offer an advantage to individuals with slowed metabolisms, such as the elderly. *Long-acting* drugs remain in the body for a longer period of time; they have a long *half-life*. They offer the advantage of a steady-state blood level of the drug, which eliminates the risk of recurrence of symptoms or withdrawal symptoms. The disadvantage of long-acting drugs is a *washout period*, a requisite period of time required between stopping the current drug and beginning to take a new drug.

Sleep apnea: (sometimes called hypersomnia-sleep apnea syndrome): a sleep disorder that causes daytime sleepiness and nighttime symptoms of restlessness and interrupted sleep. Sleep apnea is due to a partial or even complete obstruction of the upper airway. A partial blockage usually results in loud snoring or occasional sleep arousal. Complete obstruction, however, produces brief episodes of breathing stoppage. If you were taking a heavy sedative, such a stoppage could be dangerous, even fatal.

Tachycardia: an abnormally rapid heart rate, usually defined as a heart rate of over 100 beats per minute.

Tardive dyskinesia: a rare form of potentially irreversible dyskinesia. It may occur following prolonged administration of major tranquilizers. It seems to be related to age (older patients are more susceptible than younger ones) and, to a lesser degree, to sex (females are more susceptible than males). Patients with mood disorders (such as manic disorders) appear to be particularly vulnerable when treated with certain psychiatric drugs. Though highly debatable, published figures place the incidence of tardive dyskinesia as high as 10 to 20 percent of all patients on major tranquilizers, with African Americans perhaps being at greater risk for tardive dyskinesia.

Therapeutic index: the ratio of the middle dose of a drug that would be lethal versus its middle dose that would make it effective. A therapeutic index looks like this:

lethal dose: 50 percent
effective dose: 50 percent

Therapeutic window: the dose range within which a drug remains effective. Outside these limits, too little of the drug would be ineffective and too much of the drug would be redundant. Any change of dosage would produce little change or improvement.

Washout period: a period of time following the termination of certain long-lasting drugs during which the body rids itself of any traces of the drug. During this period, many other drugs cannot be taken. A washout period may vary from one to two weeks, depending upon the drug involved.

Weight gain: weight gained while taking specific medications. Different drugs cause weight gain for different reasons. One type of drug may act directly on the hypothalamus, which is the appetite and satiety center. People so affected may gain weight because of an increased appetite with an accompanying increased desire for carbohydrates. Other people who are vulnerable to weight gain from medication are those with an easily changed (or *labile*) system for governing appetite, or a system that experiences an increase of appetite whenever there is a chemical change in the acid-base composition of the intestine.

Index

Index